Partners of the Heart

Partners of the Heart

Vivien Thomas and His Work
with Alfred Blalock

An Autobiography by Vivien T. Thomas

PENN

University of Pennsylvania Press

Philadelphia

10 9 8 7 6 5 4 3 2 1

Published by
University of Pennsylvania Press
Philadelphia, Pennsylvania 19104-4011

Library of Congress Cataloging-in-Publication Data

Thomas, Vivien T., 1910–
    Partners of the heart : Vivien Thomas and his work with Alfred Blalock : an autobiography / by Vivien T. Thomas.
        p.   cm.
    "First paperback printing 1998" — T.p. verso.
    1985 ed. has title: Pioneering research in surgical shock and cardiovascular surgery.
    Includes bibliographical references and index.
    ISBN 0-8122-1634-2 (alk. paper)
    1. Thomas, Vivien T., 1910 —   . 2. Blalock, Alfred, 1899–1964. 3. Surgeons — Maryland — Biography. 4. Cardiovascular system — Surgery. 5. Shock. 6. Surgery, Experimental. I. Thomas, Vivien T., 1910– Pioneering research in surgical shock and cardiovascular surgery. II. Title.
    [DNLM: 1. Blalock, Alfred, 1899–1964. 2. Cardiovascular System — surgery — personal narratives.   3. Shock, Surgical — personal narratives.   4. Research — personal narratives. Not Acquired]
RD27.35.T46A38   1997
617'.092 — dc21
[B]
DNLM/DLC
for Library of Congress   97-14222
                                                                              CIP

To Clara Flanders Thomas

Contents

Foreword

It is clear, from all the detailed material he has had filed all these years, that Vivien Thomas had long planned some type of autobiography. It is a source of satisfaction to me that my prodding may have helped bring the work to fruition and that the secretarial assistance provided in Pittsburgh facilitated the project.

Dr. Thomas's book can, of course, be read at several levels. It is the record of the life, progress, and achievement of an American Negro with a remarkable character and a notable career. The book is written in the understated style and good humor that characterize its author; however, Dr. Thomas's staunch adherence to principle, the sense of his own worth and dignity, his comfortable independence can at times be as clearly discerned, even divined—so subtle the message—as we know them from daily association.

On another level the book provides an account, from an unusual perspective and by a remarkably perceptive observer, of the development of two major fields of research—the investigations into the nature of shock and the study of the operative relief of several forms of congenital heart disease—in which Thomas served for years as the uniquely gifted laboratory technician and collaborator of Dr. Alfred Blalock at Vanderbilt and Johns Hopkins. Thomas's insight into the problems, his accounts of their progressive solutions, his evaluations of the men with whom he worked, some already "arrived," others then still only medical students, are priceless primary sources of medical history. The stage for much of the book is the Hunterian Laboratory at Johns Hopkins under Alfred Blalock, when the department was at the height of a glorious renaissance, filled with men who have come to dominate the American surgical scene for the last thirty years and visited by surgeons from every part of the globe. Vivien Thomas worked with many of them and knew them all. The years marked the dawn of cardiac surgery, and Vivien Thomas was intimately involved.

Dr. Thomas's accounts of the development of the operation for relief of the tetralogy of Fallot, the operation for the relief of transposition of the great vessels, and the development of closed chest cardiac massage for the relief of cardiac arrest differ in some degree from the reports of others as well as from that notably erroneous category, "the generally accepted account." His story of the genesis of the operation for transposition also varies from the account I pieced together for *The Papers of Alfred Blalock*. Although I had arrived back from military service quite early in the blue baby work and was at Hopkins throughout the transposition work, and most, if not all, of the various phases of the closed chest massage work, when I collected material with reference to the tetralogy work and the transposition work, I began to despair of ever being able to determine precisely what took place, however much information I obtained directly from the principal actors. Thus in the preface to my own attempt at serious surgical history, *A Century of Surgery*, I felt constrained to say that "it is apparent to most historians that historical truth is difficult to arrive at, and in fact may not exist." While my conviction stands, we can be sure that we are here given the considered account of an intelligent and accurate observer who was himself a prime participant.

Let it here be stated for the record that this is entirely Vivien Thomas's book. The organization is his, the language is his, the accounts are his. I saw the manuscript in its various stages and contributed mainly in encouraging the author to go into more detail, provide more background, yield to the temptation to tell stories and supply illustrations. Medical science has been Vivien Thomas's life, so it is understandable that it is the focus of his book. The same intelligence and analytic cast of mind exemplified in his life in the laboratory and hospital permeate his writing.

Mark M. Ravitch, M.D.

Preface

During my career I gave little thought to writing my autobiography or memoirs. However, as the years rolled on and my life and my earlier activities became more and more public, I inevitably found myself thinking over the record of years past.

The suggestion that I write an autobiography first came from Dr. Mark M. Ravitch, who edited *The Papers of Alfred Blalock* in 1966. He wanted to know more about the relationship between Dr. Blalock and me. Dr. Richard T. Shackelford, Professor Emeritus of Surgery at Hopkins, also encouraged me to tell the story of what I had been doing all the years I had been at Hopkins. The presentation of my portrait in 1971 gave some incentive and Dr. Ravitch took full advantage of the event to launch a relentless campaign insisting that I begin writing. I was hesitant and somewhat reluctant, but a greater incentive came with the awarding of an honorary degree by Johns Hopkins University in 1976. I had never sought publicity concerning my work and had always taken my activity in life as a purely personal matter, yet now I began asking myself questions: Was my story worth the effort? Would others really be interested? If I wrote, what would I write? And—not least of all—how would I tell it? Indeed I had written little more than the notes and descriptions of experimental laboratory procedures.

What finally convinced me to take up the task was my recognition of the uniqueness of my position. A nonprofessional, I had begun working with Dr. Blalock early in his career at Vanderbilt and thus had been deeply involved in research leading to historic developments in medicine and had become associated with many men who accomplished so much in that field. I lacked the formal education and training needed to become an instructor in surgery or an administrator of a research facility, yet I served in both capacities.

I deliberately postponed this work until my retirement at which time I could write at leisure, or so I thought. Once involved in writing, I found I had committed myself to an almost full-time job. I began with old files, notes, and the two-volume *Papers of Alfred Blalock*. Reminiscing about the research in which I participated, the people with whom I have been associated, the events and experiences of the years past has been a pleasant undertaking. However, recalling and recounting accurately over forty-nine years in medical research laboratories was frequently an arduous and tedious task. Many of those with whom I have been associated very closely are not mentioned here. To any who may feel slighted, I offer my sincere apology. Presented here, to the best of my ability, are only some of the highlights of those years.

Acknowledgments

I am deeply indebted to Dr. Mark M. Ravitch, my mentor, for his encouragement and prodding (often needed). Without his guidance and patience these pages might not have been written. I am also indebted to his office staff, especially Mrs. Mary Beth Madalinsky and Mrs. Ruth Jacobson, for performing the yeoman's task of typing my manuscript with all of its revisions and additions. I wish to thank Mr. Leon Schlossberg for illustrations and pen sketches that did not appear in original publications and Dr. Ransom Buchholz for furnishing many pictures of the Vanderbilt years. Dr. Joseph W. Beard's teaching and indoctrination stimulated my interest and greatly influenced me in remaining in the field of medical research.

I wish to thank my niece, Valeria T. Spann, for critical reading and my daughter, Theodosia P. Rasberry, for the typing of some of the preliminary manuscript.

Last but not least, my expression of appreciation and my apologies go to my wife, Clara, often neglected, for bearing with me while I spent less time with her during the preparation of this manuscript than I had during my years of regular employment.

Part One

The Vanderbilt Years

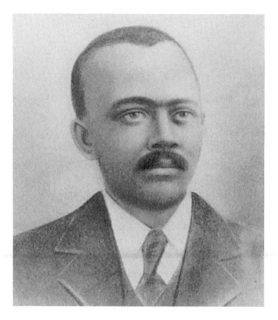

William Maceo Thomas

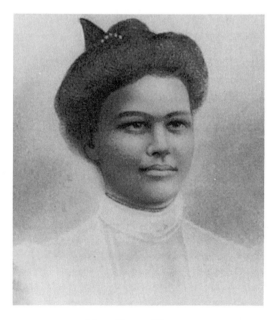

Mary Eaton Thomas

1

In 1903 William Maceo Thomas married Mary Eaton. They made their home in Lake Providence, a small town in the northeastern corner of Louisiana, not too far from the Mississippi River. It was there that their fourth child, Vivien Theodore Thomas, was born on August 29, 1910. The name given came about rather naturally; still neither of my parents ever denied my own version of the story that, since their oldest child was a girl and the next two children boys, the little girl who would surely come as the fourth was already named. I told my story in their presence while still a child and in later years on numerous occasions, much to the amusement of my father. My mother, who was more reserved and serious, didn't find the tale humorous, but I was never reprimanded for its telling.

Each spring the small community in which we lived fell victim to the flooding Mississippi. Even though the town was not inundated, communication with the outside world was possible only by small boats or canoes. "Water, water, everywhere but not a drop to drink." It was all contaminated. Most of the residents fled, only to return when the waters receded.

My parents finally grew tired of either fighting or running and in 1912 decided to move to higher ground. They settled in Nashville, in middle Tennessee, where a fifth and last child was born, the little girl they had expected three years earlier.

Besides being the capital city, Nashville was also quite an educational center. Along with a very good public school system, the city held several schools of higher education for Negroes including Fisk University, a nonsectarian school, and Meharry Medical College, one of the two medical schools in the entire country to which qualified Negroes could be assured admission for training as medical doctors. (The other was Howard University School of Medicine, in Washington, D.C.) There was also Tennessee Agricultural and Industrial State Normal School. This school was upgraded to a college in the mid-twenties and received university status many years later. Walden College was run by the Methodist church, and there were several other smaller normal and business schools. The city possessed numerous schools of higher learning for the white population, the most outstanding of which was Vanderbilt University. In addition, Nashville boasted the only exact replica of the Greek Parthenon.

The city was also a crossroad for transportation. Its three railroads, the Nashville, Chattanooga, and Saint Louis (NC & St L); the Louisville and Nashville (L & N); and the smaller Tennessee Central (TC), served traffic between North and South, East and West. Moreover, the city is situated on the Cumberland River, a navigable river, which in those days carried an appreciable amount of cargo to and from other ports along the Tennessee, Ohio, and Mississippi rivers.

Nashville had both light and heavy industry. In addition to two daily newspapers, *The Tennessean* and *The Nashville Banner*, the city held the publishing houses of three major religious organizations, the Southern Baptist Church, the Methodist Church, South, and the National Baptist Church (Negro). Negroes owned and operated two banking institutions, the Citizens Savings Bank and Trust Company and the Peoples Bank.

The majority of the Negro population occupied a large portion of the northwest section of the city extending well into the suburbs far beyond the city limits. Fisk University was in this area. Tennessee State Normal was located outside the city in Davidson County. My parents had evidently moved to Nashville at an opportune time. My father, a carpenter and contractor, must have found work plentiful for, before I was of school age, he had purchased a plot of land and had built a house on it. (The house was demolished around 1970 to make way for an expanding Meharry Medical College which had moved into the area in 1932.) The plot contained three city lots and measured 165 feet by 150 feet. This was over half an acre and provided ample garden space, which was taken full advantage of as the years passed.

My mother and father raised the five of us in this house. Our father worked endlessly to supply the family needs. He had a great sense of humor and we children often attempted to take advantage of this characteristic. He was considerate and generally indulgent but lost no time in letting us know that he and our mother were the authorities whose rules were to be obeyed.

My mother, who was an excellent seamstress, took very good care of us. She made all of the clothes for the girls and, when we boys were growing up, she made our shirts, pants, and suits. She also had the endless task of feeding all of us. When we were teenagers, we three boys would eat all the food in sight and as a result, if for any reason my father was not at the dinner table, my mother would put his food aside before we sat down to eat. Knowing how much food we devoured, I have wondered in later years why our father did not have us pay something toward the grocery bill. He referred to us as the "wrecking crew" where food was concerned.

Our home was situated equidistant from two elementary, or grammar, schools (first through eighth grades) and only two blocks from the

Fisk University campus. Pearl High School, the city high school for Negroes, was seven blocks away.

The age requirements to enter the public schools was seven years, too old to please my parents. Thus at age six, I was sent to kindergarten at Fisk University, where teacher-training courses were offered to their students. The following year I was sent to the public schools, where I remained until graduation from high school in 1929.

The teachers in the public schools were concerned and dedicated. They were determined that children would learn whatever they were supposed to learn while attending their classes. By today's standards, there was an almost unbelievable cooperation between parents and teachers. Teachers would contact parents, parents would contact teachers. Discussions might concern class work, cooperation of the pupil, areas where the pupil needed more help, effort put forth by the pupil to learn, home assignments, and the like. Discipline was seldom a school problem; it was taken care of at home. There were no habitually disruptive pupils in the classrooms. They simply were not tolerated.

The teachers began to foster a competitive spirit among the pupils in grade school by the use of simple things like spelling bees. No one wanted to be at the foot of the line. Everyone wanted to be on the honor roll or have gold stars beside his or her name, posted in one corner of the blackboard.

We were not different from any other children, but we were encouraged, motivated, and stimulated by both parents and teachers. We were mischievous, but we had both parents and teachers to keep us in line. Peer pressure and the fear of ostracism were also very effective deterrents to misconduct. It would be quite uncomfortable to have no one to talk to at lunch or recess period or no one to walk home with. Our parents took time to let us know, in no uncertain terms, what was expected of us, and we in turn made every effort to live up to their expectations. Teachers had no assistants in their classrooms, nor did they need them. Their assistants were the parents of the pupils. From parents and teachers, we learned to recognize and respect authority. Although the organization was not formal as it is today, this was the Parent-Teacher Association, and it worked. In grade school, even the principal of the school would get involved, walking to visit parents in the neighborhood. Notable among these was Ford Green, the principal of one of the schools I attended. Everyone knew, loved, respected, and cooperated with him. Ultimately, when a school was built to replace the one at which he had served for many years, the new school was very appropriately named the Ford Green Elementary School. He considered every child in his school as his own.

I attended Pearl High School, where the plant, the curriculum, and the teachers were very good. Indeed, the teachers seemed to have been hand-picked for their individual positions. They knew their subjects and their students and they knew how to teach. The academic curriculum included the standard high school courses: languages (English, Latin, French), mathematics (higher arithmetic, algebra, and geometry), history (American, modern, and ancient), and the sciences (general, biology, chemistry, physics, and geography). The school also offered vocational training. These courses were considered minor and were elective, the sessions for each class group being held for a half-day only one day a week. There were also elective courses in typing and shorthand, and, of course, there were glee clubs, choruses, a band, and a football team. I took full advantage of the curriculum, graduating with 18 credits (16 credits required).

My father took advantage of the propensity of boys to hammer on things and brought us up in his own trade of carpentry. Beside contracting the building of entire houses, he also took on repairs, additions to, and the remodeling of existing structures. He never kept us out of school for a day to work, but we were required to report after school hours to whatever job he had in progress. Our school hours were from 8 a.m. to 2 p.m., so we had from 3:00 to 5:30 to work. We also worked from 7 a.m. until noon on Saturdays. During the summer, daily work hours were from 7 a.m. to 5:30 p.m. I began reporting for work when I was thirteen. He started us out with nailing. Next, he would have us sawing (no electric saws) to lines he had made to measure on the lumber. The day would soon come when we were doing our own measuring, making our own lines, sawing, and nailing. By a gradual process we went on to finish and trim work, learning to fit and hang doors, installing locks on them, and putting in inside stairways and bannisters. As he had done with my brothers, my father had me working almost independently by the time I was sixteen years old. Work always seemed plentiful.

In addition to teaching us a trade, my father also taught us the economics of life—the fact that nothing in life is completely free. From the first time I went on a job with him, there was always an hourly rate of pay. If we were fifteen minutes late one day during a week, he would deduct it from our pay on Saturday. Of whatever amount we received, when giving it to us, he would always say, "Don't forget to give your mother something [the amount was never specified] for cooking for you and doing your laundry." He never collected anything for room and board; however, we were strictly on our own as far as our clothes and shoes were concerned. No one ever bought any wearing apparel for me after I was fourteen years old.

Working after school left little time for sports, only sandlot baseball in the summer on the corner lot a half-block away. As a result, I never became an avid sports fan. In high school, pep meetings only provided an opportunity to put in a few additional hours of work. But I was not alone; many of my classmates were doing the same.

Summertime, when schools were not in session, was a bonanza. Since we were able to work all day during these months, we could earn enough money to buy a good supply of clothes for the next school year and with luck save a few dollars. Upon graduation from high school in 1929, I thought it would be to my advantage to take a full-time job. I hoped to do other small jobs on the side and thereby save money for school.

Each summer Fisk University hired additional help for the maintenance crews, including painters, carpenters, electricians, and plumbers. During summer recess, maintenance and repair work was done on the entire facility—dormitories, classroom buildings, laboratories, and faculty houses. I had no difficulty in getting on the carpenters' crew. My family was fairly well known in the trade, and I had the reputations of my father and two brothers in my favor. At eighteen, I should be able to measure up to any situation and do anything in the field.

Mr. Elders, my foreman, knew my father well, and I had known him since I was a small boy. He was already well up into his late sixties or early seventies and could easily have been my grandfather. On my first day he sent me out with one of the older carpenters. The next morning he took me to one of the faculty houses. The inside of the house was beautiful. He showed me several things that I was to do. Included was the replacement of one piece of worn flooring in the living room near an archway into the dining room, the most conspicuous place in the room. He told me where I would find the reclaimed hardwood flooring which was stored near the central shop. This used flooring had been saved for just such situations. I was to remove the worn piece of flooring and match the color and grain to the remaining floor. Shortly after noon Mr. Elders came by to inspect. He took one look at the floor and said, "Thomas, that won't do. I can tell you put it in." Without another word, he turned and left the house. I was stung, but I replaced the piece of flooring. This time I could barely discern which piece I had put in. I worked at this same house the next two days, but Mr. Elders did not stop by again. Several days later, walking along with him to another job site, he said to me, "Thomas, you could have fixed that floor right in the first place." I knew I had already learned the lesson which I still remember and try to adhere to: whatever you do, always do your best; otherwise it might show up to haunt or embarrass you. I had spent the entire morning replacing one piece of flooring, so to make up for some of the lost time I worked for over an hour overtime.

Most of the summer Mr. Elders had me working alone and seldom came on an assignment to inspect. I learned from the other men that he did most of his inspecting before we came on the job in the morning or after we had left in late afternoon. I never had to repeat or redo another assignment.

Near the end of the summer, on the Friday before what we estimated would be our cut-off week, Mr. Elders came out of his office into the shop. He passed out pay envelopes to everyone except me and had me follow him into the office. For once he felt like talking (he was a man of few words) and gave me a little lecture to the effect that he had been in carpentry all his life and knew how long it took to do any job because he had done all of them. He said he was sure the other men had been dragging their feet, stretching jobs longer than was necessary to complete them. He had originally planned to keep all four of us on for another two weeks, but he said he could not and would not stand over any grown man to keep him working. He told me he was letting the other extra men go and was keeping me on until at least Christmas, possibly longer. I couldn't say anything except to thank him.

It was still about two weeks before Tennessee State College would be opening. Hoping to begin in the fall, I had bought a sufficient supply of clothes and shoes (shoes were all important because of the two-and-a-half-mile walk from our house to the campus), and had saved money for tuition and books. Still, I was not sure if I had sufficient funds for both tuition and for any additional books that might be required in February. Now that I was being offered the opportunity to work on through the fall, I believed that I could earn enough to register mid-year in February.

As my future turned out, the decision to continue working was possibly the most critical choice I ever made. Arguments can still be made on both sides but, at the time, only one thing was certain and that was that I had no financial backing or support to further my education. With the seasonal slowdown in construction and the collapse of the stock market in October, my job was terminated, too late to register for school. During the months that followed, only occasional small jobs were available and I found myself helping in the support of the household. But I remained determined that, regardless of what happened, the money I had saved for school would not be used for any other purpose. The immediate outlook was so poor that I decided that I was going to find a job and that I would not be choosey about the nature of that job. There had to be something beside carpentry that I could do.

2

Early in February 1930, I asked Charles Manlove, a very close friend of mine with whom I had grown up, if there were any openings for jobs at Vanderbilt University, where he was employed. He worked for Dr. Ernest W. Goodpasture in the Department of Bacteriology. I explained the situation I was in and the freeze I had put on my money. Charles told me that he knew of a job opening with Dr. Blalock at the school, but he said he understood the guy was "hell" to get along with and didn't think I'd be able to work with him. I told him that things were so tight I'd have to take my chances; I had to have some source of income.

The next morning, February 10, 1930, Charles and I went to the Medical School. We found that Dr. Blalock was scheduled in the operating room that morning, so Charles took me to the bacteriology laboratory in which he worked, preparing sterile culture media which at that time were not commercially available for the hospital and laboratory. We returned to the Experimental Surgery Laboratory around 11 a.m. When we arrived, Dr. Blalock was crossing the hall on the way to his office with a Coca Cola in his hand. Charles introduced me to Dr. Alfred Blalock at the doorway. Since Charles had told me that he was in charge of the laboratory, I expected, at the least, a mature, middle-aged person. Instead, Dr. Blalock looked more like a college senior or a medical school student. He was very cordial and polite. He thanked Charles for bringing me and invited me into his office, which was actually an individual laboratory. It held a desk, a swivel chair, two laboratory stools, a wooden animal operating table placed in front of a sink, and three pieces of apparatus (see fig. 1). I later learned that the pieces of equipment mounted on the workbench which ran across the laboratory beneath the windows were Van Slyke-Neill blood gas manometers. The apparatus on a wooden table in the corner by the sink was a Benedict-Roth spirometer. Dr. Blalock offered me a seat on one of the stools and he sat on the other, drinking his Coke and smoking.

His manner was very easygoing, quiet but serious. He first asked me if I had finished high school. He then asked if I had plans to go back to school. When I answered in the affirmative, he wanted to know why I was not then in school. I told him of my financial situation, that I would have to work my way through school. He asked what I would do if I was able to finish college, and I told him I would like to go on to medical school.

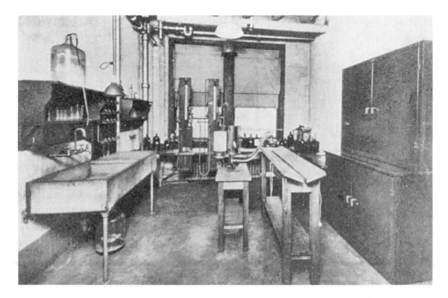

Fig. 1.   Dr. Blalock's laboratory, where his original work on shock was done. A Benedict-Roth spirometer is on the instrument table (center of room). Two Van Slyke blood-gas manometers are mounted vertically on the counter beneath the left window. From Brooks, B., Methods and Problems of Medical Education, *13th ser. New York: The Rockefeller Foundation, 1929, with permission.*

Had I worked while I was in high school? I told him of my apprenticeship with my father and how I had worked since. He then inquired about the other members of my family, how many sisters and brothers I had and their status and education. My older sister, Olga, had married and moved out of town the year before. My older brother, Harold, five years my senior, had worked his way through three years at Fisk University. After high school my other brother, Maceo, had become a carpenter, and my younger sister, Melba, was still in high school. The doctor also asked where we lived and whether my mother worked. He smiled when I said that she had worked hard—raising us—but not quite so hard anymore.

Dr. Blalock then went on to describe his situation, the type of person he was looking for, and what he expected of him. Even though I did not fully appreciate it at the time, he already knew exactly what he wanted. Essentially this is what he said to me: "As time goes on, I'm getting more and more involved with patients and hospital duties. I want to carry on my research and laboratory work and I want someone in the laboratory whom I can teach to do anything I can do and maybe do things I can't do. There are a lot of things that haven't been done. I want someone who can get to the point that he can do things on his own even though I may not be around."

He told me of the type of work he was doing and took me across the hall into the laboratory where most of the experimental surgery research was carried out. This laboratory was a large area that could accommodate eight animal operating tables, although not all of them were then in place. An autoclave was free standing at one wall with two large sterilizers alongside. A black-topped laboratory workbench ran the entire length of the room beneath the large windows opposite the entry door (see fig. 2).

Dr. Blalock introduced me to the laboratory help, Samuel Waters and Isaac Bodie. He had an acute experiment in progress in one corner of the laboratory. Apparently I was showing interest, because he went into great detail to explain to me what was being done, how it was being done, and why it was being done, and generally outlined the project he was working on.

Although very much interested in and impressed by what he was showing and telling me about his work, I was reluctant to accept the starting pay of $12 per week. This was only about two-thirds of the $20 per week I had been earning the previous summer as a carpenter. I did not really understand the economy of the country or appreciate the meaning of the economic collapse we were experiencing. To me the job was a stopgap measure to get me through the cold winter months. When warm weather arrived in the spring, I intended to go back to the Fisk University maintenance crew or out on my own to earn enough money to start school in the fall. The doctor did, however, make what I considered a promise of a raise in pay in three or four months.

After Dr. Blalock left, I stayed around the laboratory observing and asking questions. Soon after lunch time, Isaac brought in a dog from the animal quarters and he and Sam prepared and anesthetized him for an aseptic operation that was going to be performed by one of the other doctors. I watched as the doctor prepared and draped the site and then began the operation.

Sam and Isaac painted a fairly nice picture of the job and of Dr. Blalock. Their assessments of Dr. Blalock did not exactly coincide with what Charles had said, but I took into account the fact that they already worked for him and that they were not likely to give anyone a pessimistic or gloomy view of their boss or of their job. When asked directly how he was to get along with, their reply was "He's all right." I was very much interested in what was going on in the laboratory. I had also been favorably impressed by Dr. Blalock and his friendly, relaxed, and informal manner in the interview and by the amount of time he spent explaining his experiment to me. He did not strike me as being so superior that we could not or would not get along and when he returned later to check on his experiment, I told him I would try the job.

The next morning I came in for work. Dr. Blalock was there and I helped him as best I could to get his experiment started. He directed my every move. The first task was to weigh the dog and calculate the amount of barbital sodium that would be required to anesthetize him. He had me do the calculation according to the milligram per kilogram formula he gave me, and then weigh out the drug accordingly. Then came the giving of the drug. With the help of Sam, the animal was restrained on his back on the operating table. I was surprised how easily this was accomplished with Sam talking to him. Dr. Blalock injected Novocain about the femoral vessels, cut down and exposed the femoral vein, tied it off with silk, inserted a glass cannula (tube) into it through a small incision, and tied the cannula in place. Rubber tubing led from the cannula to a 50 ml.

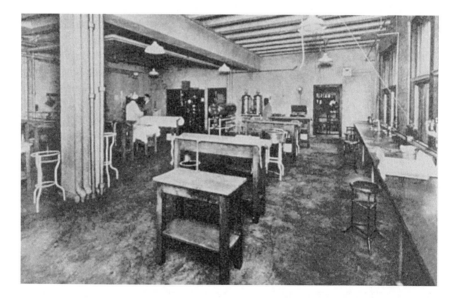

Fig. 2.   *General operating room of the experimental-surgery laboratory where classes were also held. Along far wall at center is a free-standing autoclave. The two large upright cylinders are water sterilizers. Near the doorway is a steam-heated instrument sterilizer. On the work table at right is a metric scale for weighing animals. A drum for sterile linen is on a stand partially hidden by the first operating table. Samuel Waters (with white cap) is in background with Dr. George Johnson. Isaac Bodie is near water sterilizers. Scrub sinks (not shown) are on wall to left.* From Brooks, B., Methods and Problems of Medical Education, *13th ser.* New York: The Rockefeller Foundation, *1929, with permission.*

glass burette. The barbital, dissolved in normal saline solution, was administered by being slowly poured into the burette. The animal was removed from the table and placed on the floor, where it took a little over half an hour for the anesthetic to become fully effective. During this waiting period, the equipment and apparatus for the experiment was set up. The main part of this, as I recall, was a mercury manometer and a smoked drum for recording blood pressure. When the animal was asleep, he was placed back on the table and connected to the blood pressure apparatus. This required the insertion of another glass cannula in the femoral artery. Dr. Blalock then went on with the experiment proper.

At the end of the day's work, he told me that we would do another experiment the next day and that I could come in and put the animal to sleep and get it set up. I was speechless. During my employment interview, he had told me that he wanted someone he could teach to do things. Had I gotten my first lesson and was I now expected to perform? After he left, I asked Sam and he told me, "Sure he expects you to do it; he won't show you but once." I really felt that I was on the spot. This was the first time I had even seen surgical instruments and now I was expected to use them.

The next morning with Sam's help (and moral support) I put the animal to sleep, replaced him on the table, and was in the process of putting in the arterial cannula when Dr. Blalock came into the laboratory. He was very pleasant, and after asking if I had had any difficulty, he helped me to finish putting in the arterial cannula. We then went on with the experiment. This process continued on a daily basis as he showed and told me more and more of what to do and how to do it. Two or three weeks passed and then one day he said he would be busy until such and such a time the following morning, so suppose I just went ahead without him and he would come in as soon as he was free. After the first day's experience, I had had no doubt in my mind that this type of thing would happen, so I had been putting forth every effort to observe and learn everything that was to be done. I had at times been left alone with an experiment for several hours during the day, but this was the first time I would be starting out alone.

After four or five weeks I never knew in what part of any particular experiment Dr. Blalock would participate. He would come in at any time, stay varying lengths of time, and check to see that I was doing everything right. He would ask some questions about an observation, then check the notes. If it was not there, he would tell me to write things down. "Keep your eyes open and write things down." On each occasion he repeated this four or five times in a singsong fashion. There was only one time of day when I could be certain that he would be present. That was at the time of the autopsy.

These experiments were a continuation of his studies on experimental shock. His paper "Experimental Shock: The Cause of the Low Blood Pressure Produced by Muscle Injury"[1] was already in press. Dogs, deeply anesthetized with sodium barbital, were used in all of the experiments. One of the posterior extremities was traumatized by being struck repeatedly with a hammer. From the beginning I enjoyed putting the animals to sleep, doing the cannulations, and generally setting up the experiments. Fortunately Dr. Blalock had explained the need for these experiments in such detail that I soon overcame my reluctance to inflict the trauma. Over a period of hours, the leg would swell and the blood pressure would fall; that is, the animal would go into shock.

Dr. Blalock contended that the fluid lost into the injured extremity was sufficient by itself to produce the low blood pressure or shock. Therefore, the amount of fluid in the injured extremity had to be determined. This was accomplished by comparing the weights of the injured and the opposite uninjured extremity. The difference between the weights of the two represented the fluid loss.

Dr. Blalock had already shown that the method of performing a high amputation of the posterior extremities used by other investigators did not give a true measure of the fluid loss. He had developed his own method of determining fluid loss by sectioning the body at mid-abdomen and bisecting the pelvis and lower spine longitudinally. This method, when carefully executed, would give an accurate differential between the weights of the two hind quarters (see fig. 3). Dr. Blalock was almost religious in seeing to it that the procedure was performed in accordance with his technique. I would assist him in performing the bisection one day and he would assist me the next, until he was confident I was performing it as he would himself. By today's standards and procedures, these experiments were all relatively simple, almost crude, but he was able to prove his point.

One morning Dr. Blalock came into the laboratory just as the animal was being placed on the table after having been put to sleep. He noticed that there was no cut-down and cannula in the femoral vein and inquired as to how I had put him to sleep. I told him that Tom had shown me how to give the barbital with a large hypodermic needle and a 50 cc. syringe. He smiled and said, "Tom is smart; he can teach you a lot of things." Tom Brooks was the laboratory technician to Dr. Blalock's longtime friend and colleague Dr. Tinsley R. Harrison.

The help in the Experimental Surgery Laboratory, as it was called, consisted of the two men I have already mentioned—Samuel Waters, in his late fifties, and Isaac Bodie, in his mid-sixties. Sam was the senior in years of service and was the responsible person, usually receiving the or-

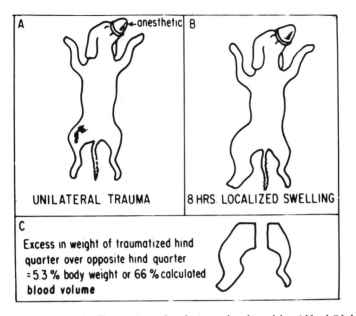

Fig. 3.   Diagrammatic illustration of technique developed by Alfred Blalock in demonstrating the pathogenesis of traumatic shock. Note that simple amputation at the hip would not recover all fluid lost in the tissue. From Sabiston, C., Jr., Alfred Blalock, Annals of Surgery 188(3): 255, September 1978, with permission.

ders from any of the investigators who scheduled work in the laboratory. He was the one who saw to it that things were done. Isaac was essentially Sam's helper. Their duties were to get animals from their quarters, put them on the operating table, and prepare them for whatever procedure was to be carried out. If anesthesia was to be administered intravenously, it was the responsibility of the investigator. If it was to be inhalation ether, which was used for chronic or survival procedures, it was administered by Sam or Isaac. Preoperatively, morphine and atropine were always administered subcutaneously for sedation. Sam and Isaac were also responsible for setting up and sterilizing the surgical instruments, for cleaning the instruments after each procedure, and for the preparation and sterilization of linen supplies. Prefolded gauze sponges were not available commercially then and sponges had to be cut and folded from bolts of gauze. This consumed a considerable amount of time and the two men would carry out the task on the workbench in the operating room even while various procedures were in progress. They also took care of all housekeeping chores, and the disposition of waste and dead animals in the incinerator, which was located in another part of the building. Sam kept a wad of chewing tobacco in his mouth at all times. For several months I thought he had a tumor of his left jaw.

There were several members of the full-time surgical staff who had research projects going in this large laboratory, but most of them worked only once or twice a week for two or three hours. Among them were Dr. Isaac Biggers, a thoracic surgeon who later went to the Medical College of Virginia as Professor and Chairman of the Department of Surgery; Dr. Beverly Douglas, a plastic surgeon; Dr. Eugene Regen, who became Chairman of the Department of Orthopedic Surgery; Dr. George Johnson, a general surgeon who had succeeded Dr. Blalock as surgical resident; and Dr. Edward Cox, a gynecologist.

Dr. Cobb Pilcher, who was to finish the surgical residency in 1932, stayed on the full-time staff specializing in neurosurgery, a relatively young field of surgery, and also began working in the laboratory. In 1940–41 Dr. Pilcher was involved in testing the effectiveness of the new sulfa drugs in combating infection on the surface and in the lobes of the brain in dogs. He was looking for a possible treatment of head wounds in the war raging in Europe. He ultimately became Chairman of the Department of Neurosurgery at Vanderbilt.

Things went very smoothly in the laboratory for about two months. We had settled down to what I considered a good working relationship. Then one morning it happened. Something went wrong, I no longer recall what, but I made some error. Dr. Blalock sounded off like a child throwing a temper tantrum. The profanity he used would have made the proverbial sailor proud of him. I just stood there looking at him. When he finished his tirade, he went to the walk-in refrigerator, got a Coca Cola, which he kept by the case, and left. When he had gone, I asked Sam how often that sort of thing happened. Sam told me it could happen any morning Dr. Blalock had had a "bad night." Remembering what Charles had said about getting along with him, I went to the locker room and changed clothes, then went across the hall to Dr. Blalock's laboratory office. I knew he would be there drinking his Coke and reading or writing. When I walked in, he looked up and asked what was the matter; he actually acted surprised, as if nothing had happened. I told him that he could just pay me off, that I was trying but if it was going to be like this every time I made a mistake and I couldn't please him, my staying around would only cause trouble. I said that I had not been brought up to take or use the kind of language he had used across the hall. He apologized, saying that he had lost his temper, that he would watch his language, and asked me to go back to work. Returning to the laboratory, I told Sam what had been said. Sam laughed and answered, "Just watch, he'll do the same thing again." I said if he did, he wouldn't see me again until the next payday, when I would come for my money. But Dr. Blalock kept his word for the next thirty-four years, even though I made mistakes. We had occasional disagreements and sometimes almost heated discussions. But neither of us ever hesitated to let the other know, in a straightforward man-to-man manner, what he thought or how he felt, whether it concerned research or, in later years, the administration of the laboratory. In retrospect, I think this incident set the stage for what I consider our mutual respect throughout the years.

Sam Waters, who had been working at Vanderbilt on the old South Campus for years and had been placed in the Experimental Surgery Laboratory when the Hospital and Medical School moved into the new facilities in 1925, was there when Dr. Blalock was put in charge of the laboratory in 1927 on the completion of his surgical residency. By the time I became employed there, Sam was pretty familiar with Dr. Blalock's reputation for prowess with the ladies and for being a great party man. And he didn't hesitate to impart these "morsels of information." He also had direct experience with Dr. Blalock's actions and reactions in the laboratory on mornings after he had been out on the town. After the incident cited above, whenever Sam thought the doctor had a hangover, he would say to me, "You better watch yourself with 'that man' today." And I learned through experience that on some mornings he could be quite difficult.

Prohibition was in effect at that time and Sam had told me that Dr. Blalock kept a five- or ten-gallon charred keg of whiskey in the laboratory storeroom at all times. I was not able to verify this for months, possibly a year, until on one occasion he was having difficulty removing the bung from a ten-gallon keg and had me help him. The keg was kept on a shelf with an old gown casually tossed over it to keep it inconspicuous. I would help him to siphon off, fairly frequently, a quart at a time. He would always start the siphon himself, usually late in the afternoon near time to go home. On only two or three occasions did he offer me a drink (with Coca Cola), each time being when we were working far past 5 o'clock and everyone had left the laboratory. At nineteen or twenty I was inexperienced and took a drink only occasionally, but I didn't think it was "bad stuff." He carried the only key on the floor to the storeroom in his pocket, usually loose, along with pocket change. If anything was needed from the storeroom, he would have to be found or we would have to wait for his return to the laboratory. The only other key to the storeroom was in the office of Dr. Barney Brooks, Professor and Chief of Surgery.

Although Dr. Blalock had his "bad nights," as Sam referred to them, he never had bad days. On an occasional morning it would be fairly obvious that he had overindulged the night before, but he never let this interfere with his daytime responsibilities and work schedule. I never saw him take a drink or even suspected that he had taken one during working hours.

I had seen the very attractive and vivacious Mary Obrien while she was working in the admitting office of the Hospital and had learned that she was Dr. Blalock's number one girlfriend. On the day of their wedding in October 1930, I picked up Dr. Blalock's car at a service station where he had left it and parked it in front of the church during the ceremony, leaving the keys in the ignition. Following the ceremony, Dr. and Mrs. Alfred Blalock marched calmly down the aisle of the church, halfway. Then they broke into a dead run as if it had been preplanned. By the time anyone reached the outside of the church, they were away on their honeymoon. No one saw them for two weeks. The society columns of the Nashville newspapers carried glowing accounts of the event describing the gorgeous gown of the bride and the beautiful dresses worn by the bridesmaids, but they omitted this little human interest side of the story, which I thought even the highest of society would have thoroughly enjoyed.

During the early months, I found it quite difficult to get along on my

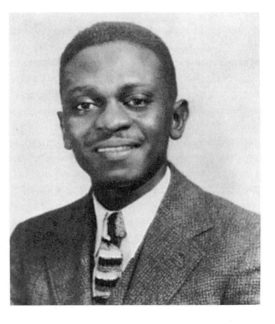

Charles H. Manlove

salary, so when they were available, I did occasional inside-the-house repair jobs for additional money. In the first part of May I reminded Dr. Blalock of his promise of a pay increase. He said he had forgotten but would look into it. After a week or more passed and he did not mention the subject, I decided to check with the foreman of the maintenance crew at Fisk University, where I had worked the previous summer, to find out what my chances of coming back were. He said, "Sure, I'll sign you in now. Go get your tools and come on back." I lived less than two blocks from the campus. I told him I could not start that day but would return the following morning.

I went to Vanderbilt to see Dr. Blalock to let him know I was leaving. I did not think it fair or right not to do this. I told him what I had done in view of the fact that he had not said anything more about an increase in my salary. He was surprised and quite upset and wanted to know how much money I would be making. When I told him that it would be the same as I had been getting the previous summer, he said, and this was the first time I noticed the whiny tone he could put in his voice, "We can't pay that kind of money. How much will you stay here for?"

I had had no idea that there could ever be any problem quitting a job and was not prepared for the negotiations that followed. He told me of all the advantages in the job I had, how nice it was working inside—you don't have to be exposed to the weather or lose time because of it. The working hours were better—8 a.m. to 5 p.m. (I could seldom leave before 6 or 6:30 p.m.), there were no strenuous physical duties to perform, a pleasant atmosphere, association with intelligent people, a paid vacation. He generally made it the most ideal job anyone could have. The only point I could make which he did not mention was that I had to make a living wage. He asked if I could and would stay around so that he could talk to Dr. Brooks, but he repeated that he did not think he would be able to get that much money for me.

After his first contact with Dr. Brooks, he came back and said Dr. Brooks did not have time to talk with him about it, that he was to see him later, but for me not to leave. After his second contact, he said he wasn't getting far with Dr. Brooks, but did not elaborate or make an offer. He had a still-later time scheduled to see him, which he did. Anyway, after some haggling, we finally settled at $17.50 per week, an amount that was well over halfway between what I was being paid and the Fisk University wage. After we had come to an agreement, he made the statement, "One day I'll have my own department and no one will be able to tell me how much I can pay people." This was in 1930. Eleven years later he had his own department, but finances would still plague him.

I began to wonder if he thought I might have the potential of being the person he was looking for, he seemed so determined to keep me on the job.

3

Up to this time, the Blalock research on shock had been relatively crude, with results obtained essentially by gross observation. The basic equipment for the mass of work he had previously turned out consisted of a mercury manometer with a float and a cross arm to record blood pressure on a smoked drum which was turned by a spring-driven motor, a Van Slyke-Neill manometric blood gas apparatus for the determination of carbon dioxide and oxygen content of the arterial and venous blood, and a Benedict-Roth spirometer to measure oxygen consumption. By figuring the difference in the oxygen content of the arterial and venous blood and knowing the oxygen uptake of the animal, the cardiac output was calculated using the Fick formula. There was also a Sahli hemoglobinometer and a metric scale to weigh the animals. In the past months, I had become fairly adept in the use of the Van Slyke apparatus, which was the most difficult to master. I was using it on an almost daily basis.

The mercury manometer was a U-shaped glass tube filled a little less than halfway with mercury. The blood pressure was obtained by connecting a piece of saline-filled rubber tubing to one side of the U-tube. The other end of the rubber tubing was then connected to a glass cannula previously inserted in the femoral or carotid artery. The pressure in the artery would be exerted upon the column of mercury and the difference in the levels of the mercury in the two columns represented the blood pressure. To record the blood pressure, a fine rod of aluminum with a hard rubber float on one end was inserted into the opposite side of the U-tube, float down. An aluminum cross arm with one end arrow-shaped was affixed to the upright rod by the use of a small piece of cork through which the two rods were passed at right angles to each other. The record proper was made on smoked, glazed paper. This paper was fastened around an open-ended drum or cylinder about six and a half inches in diameter. Inside this drum was fastened a hollow shaft which extended six to eight inches from one end. The paper was smoked by holding this shaft and rotating the drum over a kerosene lamp with a four-inch wick which gave off a cloud of dense black smoke. The hollow shaft portion of the drum with the smoked paper was then put onto the upright rod of a kymograph power unit. The motor in this unit was spring wound and could be adjusted to turn the drum at various speeds of from one inch per hour to a full turn in one minute. By placing the mercury manometer close to the smoked drum, the arrow of the crossbeam would follow the height and pulsations of the mercury column and make a continuous record of the blood pressure on the smoked paper as the cylinder turned. To create a permanent record, the paper was carefully removed and passed through a pan of dilute shellac and hung up to dry. We had extra cylinders, so Sam always kept several of them smoked and ready for use. For the shellacking, after I learned to do it, I always took care of my own. One little slip and a day's work could easily be wiped from the record. It was all an ingenious device and method in its day, but viewing it from our present electronic age of transducers, oscillographs, and built-in automatic recording devices, it seems ancient and crude.

The combined facility for Vanderbilt Hospital and the Vanderbilt University School of Medicine was constructed on the vast campus of the university and was opened in 1925. Dr. Brooks had come from Barnes Hospital, in St. Louis, to become Chairman and Surgeon-in-Chief to the institutions. At this same time, Dr. Blalock left Johns Hopkins to become Chief Resident in Surgery under Dr. Brooks, a post he was to hold for two years. Dr. Blalock had originally worked in the small individual laboratory which he had had to convert partially into office space so that he could deal with the large volume of paper work accumulated by his experimental studies. But he was not satisfied with the present arrangement of performing his experiments in the large laboratory. There were always noise, distractions, and interruptions, and there was no privacy whatsoever. One afternoon a week, work had to be scheduled to free the laboratory for a student class in operative surgery which used the area. There also were no facilities in the department to carry out studies he had in mind.

In early June workmen moved into the small individual laboratories adjoining Dr. Blalock's office. After tearing out walls, they were able to combine two and a half laboratories into one large laboratory. Here experiments could be performed on one end with sufficient space on the other for a complete chemistry laboratory (see fig. 4). Dr. Blalock now had his own private laboratory away from the hustle and bustle of the large laboratory across the hallway.

In July Dr. Joseph W. Beard became a full-time Fellow with Dr. Blalock in the laboratory. At this point the research took on a new profile. The theory that traumatic shock and the low blood pressure that accompanied it were caused by the loss of fluid from the circulation had been proven by Dr. Blalock's experiments, but the results of his studies and his conclusions were not wholly accepted. To further substantiate the validity of his findings, he now augmented his studies done essentially by gross observation with biochemical studies to determine what was being lost in the fluids that left the circulation and what changes were taking place in the circulating fluid that remained.

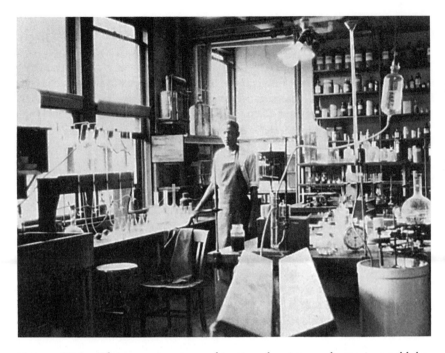

Fig. 4.   Vivien Thomas, 1931, in combination chemistry and experimental laboratory. A U-shaped mercury manometer is in direct line of operating-table trough, above which is a kymograph and smoked drum for recording blood pressure. The crock in right foreground, a constant-temperature bath with thermostat, heater, and stirrer, was assembled in the laboratory. Intravenous fluids were raised to and kept at slightly above body temperature by passing through the glass coil immersed in the water bath. On left counter is a battery of burettes for titrations of Kjeldahls and other determinations. A Barnsted still for distilled water is mounted beside window. Photo courtesy of Dr. Joseph W. Beard.

It did not take long to get the dual purpose laboratory set up with the chemicals, apparatus, and supplies necessary for the planned studies. What went on in the laboratory in the following months is best told in the following excerpts from articles by Blalock and Beard in which they described methods and gave results of some of the experiments.

EXCERPT I: Reproduced from J. W. Beard, M.D., and Alfred Blalock, M.D. *Archives of Surgery* 22:617, April 1931. Copyright 1931, American Medical Association.

METHODS

Dogs were used in all experiments. The animals were deeply anesthetized by sodium barbital (0.3 grams per kilogram of body weight given intravenously). The level of mean blood pressure was used as the criterion of the degree of shock. This was determined by placing in the carotid artery a cannula which was connected to a mercury manometer. In some instances, samples of blood were obtained from the femoral vein at the beginning and termination of the experiments and the hemoglobin was determined with a Sahli hemoglobinometer.

Samples of blood and of fluid were collected at the same time if possible. In some experiments the blood and fluid were oxalated while in others the analyses were performed on serum. The results were approximately the same whether plasma or serum was used.

The analyses of fluid and plasma or serum were carried out as follows. The sugar was determined by the method of Benedict. The sodium sulfate, which was kept as the concentrated solution, was added with the other reagents at the time of the determination. The nonprotein nitrogen was determined by the method of Folin and Wu. The chlorides were determined by the method of Whitehorn. The Gunning modification of the Kjeldahl method was used in determining the total nitrogen. One cubic centimeter of plasma or serum was the amount used in all three experiments. The mixture was heated for more than three hours. The time of distillation was forty-five minutes. One-tenth normal sulphuric acid was used for absorption of the ammonia, and the excess was titrated with one-tenth normal sodium hydroxide.

EXCERPT II: Reproduced from Alfred Blalock, M.D., and J. W. Beard, M.D. *The Journal of Clinical Investigation* 11:311, March 1932 by copyright permission of The American Society for Clinical Investigation.

Van Allen tubes were used in the hematocrit determinations. Hemoglobin estimations were performed by the method of Cohen and Smith. The control blood volume was determined by the dye method as employed by Rowntree, Brown and Roth.

The determinations of nitrogen were performed on blood serum. Albumin and globulin were separated by the use of 22.2 per cent sodium sulphate as recommended by Howe. The Gunning modification of the Kjeldahl method was employed for determining the albumin and total protein nitrogen of the serum. The total nitrogen of the urine was also determiined by this method.

I learned to do all these determinations and continued to do many of them until Dr. Blalock engaged a chemistry technician at Hopkins in 1943.

In these studies on experimental shock, the composition of the blood and of the fluid that escapes from the bloodstream after mild trauma to an extremity, after trauma to the intestine, and after burns were determined. Samples of the fluid lost from the circulation after mild trauma were obtained by making an incision in the injured area and removing sufficient subcutaneous tissue to yield the fluid sample when centrifuged. In the experiments on intestinal trauma, the samples were collected directly from the peritoneal cavity. Dogs do not blister when burned, but there is a collection of fluid in the subcutaneous tissue. As in the collection of fluid following mild trauma to an extremity, the samples in these experiments were obtained by making an incision and removing a sufficient amount of this edematous subcutaneous tissue to yield the fluid for analysis when centrifuged. Samples of blood were obtained from the femoral vein in all instances.

In the performance of these studies, even though he was working under the auspices and direction of Dr. Blalock, Dr. Beard took full charge of the laboratory. Conferences were held whenever Dr. Blalock came in. Dr. Beard also took charge of me and took an interest in teaching me that I still consider unusual. With the chemistry I had in high school, he taught me what chemistry was really all about. From the start I was very much interested even though I did not have the enthusiasm that he fairly exuded. There was no phase of the chemical determinations that he did not teach me. He brought in his physiology and chemistry textbooks for me to study and would tell me what to read up on. We would have what amounted to virtual class sessions. He told me that it was nice to be able to do a thing, but it was better to know why you were doing it. He impressed upon me the fact that scientific research was exacting. The results of our biochemical determinations could not fall "in the range of" as is sometimes accepted clinically. Normal ranges have been established for patients. In our lab everything had its own exact value, there were no normals established, each experiment had its own control or normal values. Many of the determinations were done in duplicate.

All of our chemical reagent solutions used in the determinations had to be made from solid, crystalline, or powder forms of the chemical or diluted from the concentrated forms of liquid chemicals. Today "certified" chemical reagents of any concentration are available commercially. We had to standardize our own. For me this was a time of hard work and study to become familiar with and use the additional apparatus and equipment and to learn all the various techniques and methods of the determinations required in the studies that followed. The volume of work each day was tremendous. Besides having an experiment in progress, the chemical analyses from the previous day's experiment were being done. And the days were long; there was no 8 a.m. to 5 p.m. during these studies. I don't know when Dr. Beard slept; I would leave him in the laboratory at 6 or 7 p.m. Dr. Blalock would often leave even later. I would find Beard there at 7:30 the next morning. Dr. Blalock spent most of his free time, from two hours to all day, in his adjoining office doing calculations longhand. Dr. Beard tried to get him to use the slide rule for the calculations, as he had taught me to do, but Dr. Blalock said he didn't trust it.

He would occasionally check our calculations longhand, and Dr. Beard and I would exchange smiles. I did not realize that enthusiasm was contagious until I found that I didn't mind if I occasionally had to cancel some social activity. I had obviously "caught" it from Dr. Beard.

The studies continued at a slower pace when Dr. Beard went back on the house staff after a year. However, he was determined to continue the work and, although he had his clinical duties to perform, he spent a tremendous amount of time in the laboratory. The telephone rang constantly for him and if he did not answer the hospital operator (and often he did not), he would be paged. This would really rile him because it was a signal to Dr. Blalock that he was neglecting his clinical duties. With the zeal he had for research, it came as no surprise when I learned several years later that he was at Duke University devoting all of his time to it.

Following Dr. Beard's first and full year in the laboratory, there was a succession of medical students who worked with us, Harwell Wilson and Bernard Weinstein the first year. They were succeeded by Rollin A. Daniel and Sam Upchurch. The latter two worked, almost alone, on one aspect of the shock problem.[2] All four of the above coauthored papers with Dr. Blalock. After graduation, Dr. Wilson received his surgical training at the University of Chicago and later became Professor and Chairman of the Department of Surgery at the University of Tennessee at Memphis. Dr. Weinstein completed his surgical training and later became Associate Clinical Professor of Surgery at Vanderbilt. Dr. Daniel graduated in 1933, completed his surgical residency at Vanderbilt in 1938, and stayed on the full-time staff working primarily in thoracic surgery. He ultimately became Professor of Clinical Surgery. Dr. Upchurch went on to become Clinical Professor of Surgery and Chief of the Department of Plastic Surgery at the University of Alabama.

Many other students worked on the Blalock team over the following years, some for a quarter, some all summer or just on "free time" during the regular school year. Of one of the students a few years later Dr. Blalock commented, "Hell, if I had the kind of money that guy has, I wouldn't be around here working and studying that hard." He went on to say he couldn't see how the man could possibly be interested in medicine and really treating the patients or have compassion for them. Dr. Blalock was proven wrong in his assessment of this particular student. His name was Dr. Rudolph Light. The scion of a family controlling a large share of the Upjohn Corporation, Dr. Light completed his residency in surgery at Vanderbilt. Maintaining his interest in medicine and research, he subsequently became Associate Professor of Surgery and Director of the Experimental Surgery Laboratory, the very laboratory Dr. Blalock had charge of. A laboratory subsequently built bears his name. He became a trustee of Vanderbilt University in 1964.

Throughout his career, Dr. Blalock took great interest in medical students who came to him concerning research. He would always encourage them, work them into his own program, get them into the program of another investigator, or occasionally allow them to do some project of their own if he did not think it too large or complicated for them to manage alone.

In 1933 he was invited to give the Fifth Annual Arthur Dean Bevan Lecture of the Chicago Surgical Society. Even though he had published the results of his most recent findings on shock, he was quite pleased and happy to be able to present his entire argument on this topic in person to this distinguished and prestigious group. This also was his first "named lecture." He chose the title "Acute circulatory failure as exemplified by shock and hemorrhage."[3] In his most recent biochemical studies, it had been shown that the fluid lost from the circulation in trauma contained life-sustaining protein and that the protein which remained in the circulation became diluted. These were important observations, protein being the substance which by osmosis attracts fluid to the circulation and holds it there. Armed with these findings, he took great care in the preparation of his presentation. He seemed to have taken the attitude that this was his big chance and that he was going to take full advantage of it.

At the time, there were several theories on the subject of shock, some of them championed by older, more established and recognized physiologists and investigators. This meant that at age thirty-four, Dr. Blalock was challenging the establishment.

I was the audience in his preparation for the address. He memorized long passages of it and I would follow him from his manuscript.

Near the time for him to deliver the address, I asked what happens if someone is proven wrong, as he was trying in his speech to prove others were. What does one say? He smiled and said that you don't say anything, you usually keep quiet. When he returned, I asked how it had gone. He smiled and said, "Very well." I assumed that at least he was satisfied with his delivery and with the reception he'd received. The invitation itself had assured him that someone was taking note of him and his work.

In his studies on shock Dr. Blalock investigated numerous approaches to its production and treatment. Muscle injury, intestinal trauma, hemorrhage, burns, and histamine had been used as methods of its production. In the treatment of shock, the effects of various solutions and fluids, crystalline and colloidal, had been studied. They were administered intravenously, subcutaneously, intraperitoneally, and by gavage or stomach tube. The fluids had included salt solution, glucose, and gum acacia in different concentrations, singly and in combination, as well as whole blood and plasma or serum. We had also studied the effects of heat and cold. These experiments, the early ones of which were relatively simple, were always well planned, meticulously executed, and carefully observed. Dr. Blalock believed in statistics and insisted on large numbers of experiments in any series of studies in order to have meaningful statistics from which he could judge and draw conclusions.

In a series of studies on the effect of cold in shock, the experiments were to be performed in a walk-in refrigerator. The refrigerator was small for a walk-in, measuring only about four feet by five feet, its entrance located in an anteroom off the large classroom area. First of all I had to measure to determine if the space would accommodate the length of an operating table. Then there would be a table or stand for the spirometer, and something would have to be worked out about space for the blood pressure-recording apparatus. There was a set of metal shelves along one side of the refrigerator with space on one shelf reserved for Dr. Blalock's case of Coca Colas. He drank four to eight a day and one had to be a distinguished visitor to be offered a bottle. It quickly became clear that it would be necessary to remove the rack of shelves. Of course Dr. Blalock wanted to know what I was going to do about his Cokes. When I told him there would be no space for them in the refrigerator with the other equipment, he left but returned about an hour later. He stood around watching while Sam, Isaac, and I finished moving the equipment into this small area. We were having quite some difficulty getting it all in and set up so that I would have sufficient space to get in to perform the experiments and take observations. Dr. Blalock had made practically no comments or suggestions, but just about the time we completed the setup he asked, "Now what are you going to do about my Cokes?" Not realizing how serious he was, I smiled and said that I didn't know. "Well, they have to go in there somewhere," he insisted. But he had it figured out. He sent Isaac to the receiving room to get a small empty cardboard box that would hold about six bottles, being specific that it could be no larger. When Isaac returned, Dr. Blalock put five Cokes in the box (that was its capacity) and personally wedged the box into a space he had spied beneath the small square table on which the spirometer was standing. He had spent at least forty-five minutes seeing to it that his Cokes would be cold when he wanted one.

One day in the early thirties, Dr. Blalock came into the laboratory with several bottles of capsules labeled Nembutal, manufactured by Abbott Laboratories. He told me that it was a barbiturate, but that it was not as profound or as long acting a drug as the barbital sodium we were using for anesthesia in the acute studies on shock. If it worked out, it might be possible to use it instead of ether as general anesthesia in chronic experiments.

He had no idea how much it would take intravenously. I was to empty the capsules, make up several concentrations of solutions, and try putting some dogs to sleep by titration. I could use some of the dogs we had operated upon for long-term experiments, our "chronic preparations," but was to be careful not to kill any of them. Going out of the door, he called back, "Don't you kill any of those dogs." Some of "those dogs," of course, already represented many hours of work and observation—all lost if they died since the experiments could not then be carried to conclusion.

It took an average of thirty minutes for the barbital sodium to have full effect. My first few dosages of the Nembutal were all underestimated; the animals were up and walking around in thirty minutes or less. By gradually increasing the dosage, I found that it required 30 milligrams per kilogram to get a good surgical anesthesia with a duration of from two hours to about three and a half hours depending upon the operative procedure. Some time later, the powdered form became available, and still later, Abbott Laboratories began supplying a clinical solution containing 50 milligrams per cubic centimeter. For ease of calculation of dosage (30 milligrams per kilogram) for our animals, our solution contained 60 milligrams per cubic centimeter. We began using it extensively for general anesthesia. I did not learn of the veterinary product until the veterinarians moved into Hopkins somewhere in the late fifties.

4

I had done or had assisted during numerous minor acute surgical procedures—cutdowns of femoral or neck vessels and the bisections of animals at autopsy during the shock studies—but the first project that I considered to involve "real surgery" was our work on the effect of adrenalectomy on cardiac output.[4] This took place during the period that Dr. Beard, although officially on the clinical service, was spending time in the laboratory. The operations were carried out with aseptic techniques and were my first experience in doing, or rather, assisting in aseptic surgical procedures—putting on a cap and mask, scrubbing up, putting on a sterile gown and gloves, and adhering to operating room techniques.

Most of these operations were performed by Dr. Blalock, usually in the afternoon while we had an acute shock experiment in progress in the chemistry laboratory. I would leave the acute experiments to scrub up and assist him. The adrenal glands, although small in size, are somewhat difficult to remove due to their anatomical location and blood supply. They lie above the kidneys on each side, just beneath the diaphragm, and are most easily approached through a posterior subcostal (flank) incision. The operations were staged, that is, the adrenal was removed on one side and the animal allowed to recover. Several weeks later, the other adrenal gland was removed and the studies began. The Van Slyke was used for oxygen determinations. Some of the late-night (9:00 or 10:00 p.m.) observations and oxygen determinations were done by Dr. Blalock. He worked as long and as hard as everyone else; it was never a matter of "You do it, I'm gone." It was "follow the leader."

Since these experiments did not occupy a full day's work, there were overlapping projects in progress at all times. One would have priority, but if some unusually interesting observation was made in one of the secondary projects, that project would likely be given priority and would be studied until some conclusions could be reached or the idea abandoned. Sometimes a short, uncomplicated project such as that on the effect of complete occlusion of the thoracic aorta[5] would be completed as a secondary project. This overlapping of projects is an example of how Dr. Blalock "never put all his eggs in one basket." If one research project completely failed, he always had another in progress.

Dr. Gunnar Nystrom, Professor of Surgery at Upsala, Sweden, was Abraham Flexner Lecturer in Surgery at Vanderbilt in 1935. He worked in the laboratory with Dr. Blalock for about two months on studies of pulmonary embolectomy.[6] At that time, relatively little was known about the length of time the major vessels, the aorta and pulmonary artery, could be safely occluded. With the little experience I had in operating, I was impressed by Dr. Nystrom's dexterity and the smoothness of his operative technique in working on these large vessels so close to the heart.

It had been known for many years that patients with kidney disorders often exhibit hypertension (high blood pressure). The condition is far less frequent than the so-called essential hypertension in which there is no discoverable organic cause. It had been established that renal hypertension could be produced experimentally by causing renal ischemia, that is, by reducing the volume of blood flowing through the kidneys. Dr. Harry Goldblatt, of Cleveland, had recently developed a technique and an instrument to accomplish this condition very consistently. The method, while reducing the blood flow through the kidneys, produces hypertension, but does not measurably reduce renal function.

Around 1935, in efforts to learn more of the etiology of the condition, Dr. Blalock teamed up with Dr. Tinsley R. Harrison. Harrison and Blalock had been roommates in medical school at Hopkins and after graduation had worked together in the laboratory there. The two doctors came to Vanderbilt at the same time, Harrison as Resident in Medicine and Blalock as Resident in Surgery. Morton F. Mason, Ph.D., joined them in the study of renal blood flow and oxygen consumption. In the studies, hypertension was produced by the Goldblatt method, reducing the flow of blood through the kidney.[7] The blood flow was measured directly by the use of a cannula devised by Harrison and Blalock (see fig. 5). It consisted of a long, polished brass tube with two rubber cuffs which formed balloons when inflated, one near the closed distal end, the other located about three inches proximal, with large perforations between the two. This cannula was passed into the external jugular vein through the superior vena cava, down through the heart, and into the inferior vena cava until the distal cuff was beyond the renal veins, thus placing the proximal cuff between the renal veins and the hepatic veins. The cuffs could be inflated with a syringe through minute indwelling copper tubing that came out of the side near the proximal end of the cannula. The inflated distal balloon would obstruct the flow of blood from the posterior extremities and lower part of the body, and the proximal balloon would occlude the cava proximal to the kidneys. Thus, only the blood from the kidney flowed into the cannula through the perforations and out through the cannula to which rubber tubing was attached. The rate of blood flow through the kidney was determined by collecting blood as it flowed from the rubber tubing into a calibrated glass cylinder and timing the volume per minute with a stopwatch. The cannula being smaller than the cava,

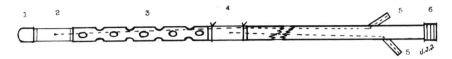

Fig. 5.   Blalock-Harrison cannula used in the crude but effective technique for direct measurement of renal blood flow. The tubing was ¼-inch-diameter polished brass, 45 cm. long. 1: Closed, rounded end. 2: Turned-down area with grooves for tying on Penrose tubing (balloons). 3: Perforations (7.5-cm. segment) for outflow of blood. 4: Penrose tubing tied in place. 5: Nipples for rubber-tubing connections to syringes to inflate balloons. Dotted lines represent small indwelling tubing through which balloons are inflated. 6: Brass sleeve to accommodate slightly larger rubber tubing through which outflow of blood is measured.

the level of the tip of the rubber collecting tube was adjusted downward, to take advantage of gravity or suction, to assure that there was no back pressure buildup in the renal veins.

During one of these experiments, Dr. Blalock was on the stopwatch, Dr. Mason collecting the blood in the cylinder, I was inflating the balloons, and Dr. Harrison was keeping the notes. At one point Dr. Mason let the tip of the rubber tubing slip and got quite a bit of blood on his pants. Dr. Harrison dutifully noted, "Mort got blood on his pants." After several more measurements had been taken, Dr. Blalock went over to where Dr. Harrison was sitting, taking notes, to compare the readings. When he saw what Dr. Harrison had written, he asked, "Why the hell did you have to write that down?" Harrison replied, "Well, Al, you know how you are about writing things down. There's a two-minute time gap and you would be wondering what happened." Everyone laughed except Dr. Blalock, for whom there was seldom anything amusing where work was involved. Dr. Harrison was just the opposite; he would always keep some light banter going. Dr. Blalock was fond of sports and occasionally would speak of something sports related, but he would always bring the conversation directly back to the research project. It was interesting to observe that two people with such different personalities and senses of humor could be and were such close friends. It was during one of these experiments that Dr. Harrison jokingly commented, "Don't let Al tell you that he had health problems because he worked so hard. He worked hard all right, but it was the things he did after leaving work that got him into trouble." He seemed to thoroughly enjoy seeing Dr. Blalock squirm.

Dr. Blalock had begun to determine cardiac output in his experimental work even before his work on shock. In these early experiments, the only apparatus available for determining the oxygen content of the blood had been the Van Slyke (long bore) apparatus which had to be shaken by hand. Dr. Blalock changed to the newer Van Slyke-Neill apparatus during the progress of the experiments on cardiac output in pneumonia in dogs, reported with Dr. Harrison in 1926.[8] In the article, he indicates the use of both kinds of apparatus. Two of a still more refined version of the Van Slyke-Neill manometric blood gas apparatus were acquired when the new Chemistry and Experimental Laboratory was set up in 1930.

The difference in the oxygen concentration of arterial blood going to the kidney and of venous blood leaving the kidney is very small. In one phase of our studies in which renal arterial flow was reduced mechanically, to produce hypertension, the determinations of the oxygen content of the blood were considered particularly critical. Dr. Harrison said that he didn't trust my oxygen determinations and Dr. Blalock said that he didn't trust Dr. Harrison's. (I really think that Dr. Harrison, intending this as one of his jokes, was actually trying to get Dr. Blalock to do the determination himself.) As a compromise, both Dr. Harrison and I did determinations on each blood sample, in duplicate. Dr. Harrison's laboratory was on the same floor as ours, but directly across a large courtyard with connecting wings of the building on each end. Dr. Blalock acted as runner and referee. He would take the syringes containing the blood samples back and forth between the two of us and collect our results on each determination. This would go on for two to three hours, at the end of which time we would all get together and compare results. Both of us were doing oxygen determinations in duplicate and our differences were almost nil. This routine continued for eight or ten experiments. Of course, on one occasion Dr. Harrison could not resist the chance to quip, "See, Al, Vivien is better than you. I know my results are right and you have never been able to check them that closely."

The experiments in the several projects carried out by Drs. Harrison and Blalock were all preplanned to the last minute detail. There was little discussion in the laboratory once an experiment was in progress. Dr. Blalock may have had it this way because otherwise there would always have been the problem of keeping Dr. Harrison from making those uncomfortable quips.

Dr. Arthur D. Grollman, at Hopkins, was also working on hypertension. He and Dr. Harrison were tackling the same phase of it, using supposedly identical methods and techniques, but getting different results. One day while we were all working together in the laboratory, Dr. Harrison told us how vigorously Dr. Grollman had tried to get him to come to Hopkins so that they could discover what Dr. Harrison was doing wrong. Dr. Harrison, on his part, was determined to get Dr. Grollman to his laboratory. He made quite an amusing story of it, saying there was no way that he could lose on his home territory and before Grollman got away he was going to show that it was Grollman who was making the mistakes. Dr. Arthur Grollman was on the faculty of Johns Hopkins until 1941, when he went to Wake Forest University School of Medicine. In 1949 he became Professor of Medicine and Chairman of the Department of Experimental Medicine at Southwestern Medical School of the University of Texas. He is best known for his work on blood volume, peritoneal dialysis, and hypertension. He retired in 1977.

When the team of Blalock and Harrison broke up in 1941, Dr. Tinsley R. Harrison went to Wake Forest University Medical School. He took James Lewis along with him as his technician. In 1946 he moved to Southwestern Medical College as Professor of Medicine and Dean of the Faculty. He returned to his native state, becoming Professor of Medicine at the Medical College of Alabama in 1949 and retiring in 1966. James went with him to Texas, but refused to leave there. Dr. Harrison told me that James had bought a farm, was involved in politics, and would probably become mayor of the town. James is now retired and resides in Seagonville, Texas.

Until about 1935, the major focus of the work in the laboratory was on the problem of shock, which we had studied from almost every conceivable angle. Numerous other projects were being done concurrently, many of which involved the setting up of chronic surgical preparations. These included studies on the effects of division of the cervical esophagus,[9] the effects of the perforation of peptic ulcers,[10] total pneumonectomy,[11] experimental production of chylothorax,[12] and many others. The results of many experiments were deemed insignificant by Dr. Blalock and never published. However, these projects involved surgical procedures from which I began to learn something of surgical techniques.

In doing these and other operative procedures, when nothing else was scheduled or when some acute experiment had been set up and was in progress, I would scrub up, prepare, and drape the anesthetized animal. When Dr. Blalock came in to scrub, he would have me begin the incision. His scheduled arrival time allowed me to judge my starting time. One day he didn't make his schedule. I waited a while, made the incision, and covered it with moist gauze. I waited some more. Ten to fifteen minutes later he came in. "Sorry. I got tied up," he said. On another day, I made the incision and waited thirty minutes. After forty-five minutes, when he still had not come, I went ahead with the procedure and slowly and painstakingly struggled on through alone. He came in just as I was ready to close the incision. After looking over what I had done, he asked who had helped me. I said no one and Sam confirmed my reply.

In the early chronic surgical procedures it became more or less routine that, unless it was practically impossible to do a procedure alone, I would assist him on a particular procedure only the first time. Usually after that, I could never be sure that he would be there. He would often come into the laboratory while I was operating and ask if I needed help. If I said I did, he would usually scrub in and assist rather than take over the procedure. If I said I did not need help, he would sometimes comment that he did not see how I could do the procedure alone. At times a medical student working with us part time might be available to assist. For times when no help was available, I had taught myself to use traction sutures and pack off with gauze sponges to get exposure. This technique worked much better than an assistant who did not understand what I was trying to accomplish. At least a traction suture anchored to the edge of an incision maintained consistent traction. Dr. Blalock would sometimes stand by and watch while I was trying to get exposure.

With the team of Blalock and Harrison, research was going full steam ahead. Since Dr. Blalock had not had a full-time postdoctoral fellow in the laboratory since Dr. Beard, the coming of Dr. Sanford E. Levy, from the University of California, in July 1936, was very welcome. The studies on renal hypertension required innumerable chronic experimental surgical preparations and, with Dr. Blalock's time in the laboratory becoming more and more limited, these preparatory procedures were mainly left to Levy and me. Dr. Blalock was almost always present when studies were done however. Since these preparatory procedures and studies were already underway when Levy joined the team, I had more experience with them and with previous experimental surgical procedures. But it was not long before Levy and I were working as a team on these experimental surgical procedures, alternating as surgeon and assistant.

To determine the effect on the blood pressure of constricting the renal artery of a completely denervated kidney, the artery, vein, and ureter had to be divided to leave no doubt about the interruption of all nerve fibers running along these structures. The circulation of the blood to and from the kidney, and the drainage of urine through the ureter had to be reestablished. Why not do this at a place where the vessels would be more easily accessible than in the normal position? Dr. Blalock decided on transplantation of the kidney to the neck.[13] Neither he, Levy, nor I had had any experience in doing vascular surgery. Dr. Blalock, however, did have a clinical case to his credit, reported in "Successful Suture of a Wound of the Ascending Aorta."[14]

This was the project on which we all three learned or taught ourselves vascular surgery. The only reference available to us was the method of Alexis Carrel, described almost thirty years before. As in the above-mentioned procedures, the brunt of the transplantation fell on Levy and me. The kidney was removed through a subcostal, flank incision, preserving the full lengths of the renal artery and vein and 5 or 6 cm. of ureter (see fig. 6). The jugular vein and carotid artery were exposed in the neck and a pocket to hold the kidney was made beneath the skin in the neck. The vessels in the neck were ligated distally and divided, with bulldog clamps occluding them proximally. By using three stay sutures to approximate and triangulate the ends of the vessels, the carotid artery was sutured to the renal artery and the jugular vein sutured to the renal vein. The bulldog clamps were then removed. The kidney was placed in the pocket beneath the skin with the renal pelvis toward the heart, thus placing the vessels in a straight line. The ureter was brought out through a stab wound in the skin. The incisions were closed with interrupted silk sutures.

Dr. Blalock and Rudolph Light were scrubbed in on some of these early transplants. The tedious and time-consuming procedure took as long as three and a half to four hours. The kidney was without circulation for as long as one and a half hours. Levy and I soon worked out a

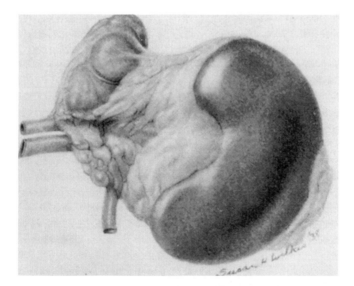

Fig. 6. This drawing shows how the transplanted adrenal gland is bound by connective tissue to the renal pedicle and the kidney. The renal artery and vein were sutured to the carotid artery and the jugular vein. The ureter was brought out through the skin and as the kidney functioned, urine dripped freely. In transplantation of the kidney alone, the adrenal gland was dissected free of the renal pedicle and left in place. From Levy, S. E., and Blalock, A.: A method for transplanting the adrenal gland of the dog with re-establishment of its blood supply, Annals of Surgery *109 : 84, January 1939, with permission.*

routine. He prepared the vessels in the neck and I removed the kidney. Then, working together to do the blood vessel suturing, we cut the overall procedure time to about one and a half hours, and the circulation to the kidney was restored in about thirty minutes.

At the very beginning of this project we encountered a big problem with the suture material. Suture material for blood vessels has to be very fine. Johnson and Johnson produced arterial sutures put up in sterile glass tubes. The fine calibre, inch-long needle worked well but the silk was twisted and would invariably fray while suturing. We were able to obtain a treated 5-0 braided silk manufactured by J. A. Deknatel and Son. When we removed the needles from the twisted silk, we found that the eye was so small we had to use a magnifying glass to thread them with the braided silk. Later we were able to thread the needles by "guessing" where the eye was.

The renal artery constricting device that Goldblatt had designed was made of silver and was supplied to Dr. Blalock by Dr. Goldblatt. The device was so small and difficult to maneuver that Goldblatt had also designed an instrument to handle it during application. Dr. Blalock was never a great one for gadgets, but he had a great liking for applying these and must have personally put on 75 to 80 percent of the numerous ones used. Sometimes, with the vessel already exposed, he would scrub in just long enough to apply the "Goldblatt Clamps," as we referred to them. I never had the impression that he didn't trust Levy or me; this just happened to be a gadget he liked.

With the idea of producing pulmonary hypertension, Dr. Blalock had us perform a series of operations in which the proximal end of the divided left subclavian artery was anastomosed to the distal end of the divided left pulmonary artery (see fig. 7). The preparations were done with the same vascular suture technique that had been used in the kidney transplantation project. Blood from the systemic circulation, at a pressure of 120 to 140 millimeters of mercury, was put into the pulmonary circulation, which normally has a pressure of 25 to 30 millimeters of mercury. Subsequent studies of these preparations revealed little or no change in the pressure in the pulmonary system, or in the wall of the pulmonary arteries.[15]

We had so much technical success with the kidney transplantation that some time later Dr. Blalock decided we should try to transplant the adrenal gland.[16] The blood supply of the adrenal gland does not have individual vessels large enough for direct anastomoses. However, the gland is so bound in and attached to the renal pedicle that it seemed reasonable to assume that it was getting a good percentage of its blood supply from the renal pedicle (see fig. 6). With this reasoning, Dr. Blalock decided to use

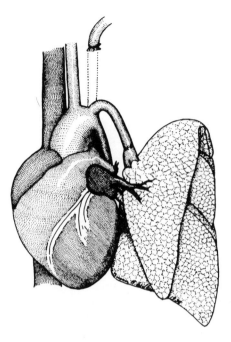

Fig. 7. Subclavian–pulmonary artery anastomosis was used experimentally at Vanderbilt in 1938 in an attempt to produce pulmonary hypertension. The vascular changes of pulmonary hypertension were not produced, but the technique was the answer to the problem of patients with the tetralogy of Fallot when several years later it was suggested that those patients needed an operation that would bring more blood to the lungs. From Levy, S. E., and Blalock, A.: Experimental observations on the effects of connecting by suture the left main pulmonary artery to the systemic circulation, Journal of Thoracic Surgery 8:525, June *1939, with permission.*

the renal vessels for the direct anastomosis, after carefully dissecting the adrenal free from its other attachments. The kidney and its pedicle, and the adrenal, were removed en masse and transplanted to the neck using the technique employed in the simple kidney transplant: viz., carotid artery to renal artery and renal vein to jugular vein. The kidneys were put in place in a pocket beneath the skin. A week to several months later, the kidney was removed without disturbing the renal vessels which nourished the adrenal gland. The rate of success of the transplantation was about 50 percent, as demonstrated by the survival of the animals when the other (right) adrenal gland was removed at a later date. Without adrenals, animals die of adrenal insufficiency from the experimentally produced Addison's Disease.

Originally, Levy was to spend one year in research as a part of his surgical residency program, but the research projects were going along so well and he was putting so much into them that Dr. Blalock asked him to stay on for a second year. He returned to the University of California to complete his surgical training, after which he joined the faculty. He subsequently changed his name to Sanford Leeds.

In 1937 Dr. Blalock told me that he was considering an offer to go to Henry Ford Hospital, as Chief of Surgery, and that if he accepted, he wanted me to go with him. I wrote my older sister, Olga T. Calhoun, who lived in Detroit, telling her of the possibility that I might be coming there. She wrote back and told me not to get my hopes too high, that Henry Ford was strictly lily white, and that it was worse than anything she had seen, even though she had grown up in the South. Some time later, Dr. Blalock said simply, "We won't be going to Detroit." He made no further comment and gave no reason for turning down the offer. It was at about this time, however, that he was given the rank of Professor of Surgery at Vanderbilt. To me this indicated that at least some of the powers-that-be were interested in keeping him at Vanderbilt. It has been said and written [17] that the position was turned down because, as my sister had suspected, I was not acceptable to them and that I was a part of a sort of package deal that Dr. Blalock had proposed.

Dr. Ralph Cressman, who was also from the University of California, succeeded Levy as a Fellow in the laboratory. He took up at least one phase of the renal hypertension studies where Levy had left off. We also worked on at least two other phases of renal hypertension during his tenure. There were also projects done on the experimental production of osteomyelitis [18] and on the effect of pulse on the flow of lymph. [19]

Even with these widely divergent subjects under study, Dr. Blalock never lost sight of the problems of shock. There were always ideas and findings which needed further investigation. Other investigators were working on it and writing about it. As a result, a series of experiments on traumatic shock were performed in an effort to determine the role of the nervous system. [20]

In mid-December 1940, for the second time in a little over three years, Dr. Blalock called me into his office to tell me that he had received an invitation to go elsewhere. This time it was to become Surgeon-in-Chief and Chairman of the Department of Surgery at Johns Hopkins. He was going for an interview the next day. In essence, he said that it was the kind of offer "one does not turn down," even though Vanderbilt offered more money. At Hopkins he would be on a straight salary, which he would not mind, except that, as head of the department, he would be the only one required to be full time and not collect fees from patients. He closed by saying, "If I accept it, and I'm sure I will, I want you to go with me." A few days before Christmas he told me that he had accepted the offer. I was to start thinking seriously about moving to Baltimore.

The volume of work had not decreased after Cressman left in mid-1939, and by this time Dr. Blalock had very little time to spend in the laboratory. Besides his regular and growing clinical, teaching, and administrative responsibilities and his ever-increasing involvement with various professional organizations, he was named to the Committee on Surgery of the National Research Council and was made Chairman of the Sub-Committee on Shock. On occasions, I would drive him to the airport in midmorning and bring his car back to the hospital, where he would pick it up that night. He would be back in the hospital and laboratory the next morning. He complained that the trips to Washington were taking him away too often, but he continued them. Since his laboratory time had almost completely disappeared, he had me find someone to help me as needed. I was able to get Andrew Manlove, a younger brother of Charles, who had recommended me for my job. Andrew was just out of high school. He had been working closely with me, setting up experiments and assisting in operative procedures for about a year when Dr. Blalock accepted the appointment at Hopkins. I immediately began to give him more responsibility and had him perform the experimental procedures so that, when I left, he would be in a position to perform, whoever the prime investigators happened to be, or whatever might be required of him. Years later, in 1953, I received a card from Dr. Thomas N. P. Johns, who had worked in the laboratory with me at Hopkins and was visiting Vanderbilt. It stated simply, "Saw Andrew operate this day." While teaching Andrew, I had no way of knowing that he was to be only the first of many surgical technicians I would train.

Andrew and I had just completed a series of procedures in which the proximal end of the divided left subclavian artery was anastomosed to the distal end of the divided left pulmonary artery, end-to-end, when Dr. Blalock accepted the call to Hopkins. These animals were to be held for long-term studies. The earlier group done by Levy and me had only been studied on a short-term basis: about four months maximum. Five of this latter group were sent to Hopkins and were studied after a long interval. The results were found to be almost insignificant.

One of the people I remember vividly from this last year at Vanderbilt was Dr. Ransom Buchholz, a Fellow in the laboratory. I recall him so clearly, not because of any great scientific discovery or any new surgical technique he developed, but because of his personality and grand sense of humor. Regardless of how difficult the problem, or how hard he was working, Buchholz always found time for the lighter side of things, some jokes or some story to tell, anything to break the strictly business atmosphere of the laboratory.

Dr. Buchholz worked with Dr. Beverly Douglas, the plastic surgeon, studying the circulation of blood in pedicle skin grafts. Buchholz was also attempting to encase a long segment of small bowel in plastic and to obstruct the segment of bowel. He hoped to demonstrate that it was the dilation of the bowel in intestinal obstruction that causes the necrosis of the mucosa, thereby proving that the Wangensteen suction was a good treatment in these cases. Even though he did not work with Dr. Blalock and me, I was able to find time to help him with the new plastic sheet; at that time it was new on the market and was quite difficult to work with. He completed his surgical residency in 1943 and went into the armed service. At the end of World War II, he returned to Vanderbilt as an Assistant Professor of Surgery for a year, and then went into private practice.

Dr. Blalock was strictly opposed to my helping anyone in the laboratory. I first learned of this around 1934–35. Dr. Blalock came into the laboratory one day and found me helping Dr. Ralph Larsen, Resident in Surgery, with something he was doing. He told me in no uncertain terms, with Larsen listening, "You are *my* technician and you are not to help anyone." I got the word but, if I knew Dr. Blalock was busy elsewhere or was out of town, I would help anyone if I had the time available. I was interested and curious about everything that went on in the laboratory. The interest and curiosity still remain with me.

5

For the eleven years I was at Vanderbilt, I had a minimum of contact with Dr. Brooks. The first time I saw him and recognized him for who he was, was around 1933. He came into the laboratory one day while I was operating alone, with Sam giving the anesthesia. He came over and stood a little behind me and looked on for a minute or two. I continued with whatever procedure I was doing. Since he did not say anything, I more or less ignored him. He walked away, clearing his throat. After he left, I asked Sam who he was, and Sam told me it was Dr. Brooks. Since Southerners usually exchange greetings in the morning, I asked if he had seen him earlier in the morning. When Sam said he had not, I asked why they didn't speak. Sam replied, "He doesn't speak to me, so I don't speak to him." He ended any further discussion by saying, "He's just that way, so I don't bother him."

My next contact with Dr. Brooks was about a year later. The purchasing of the laboratory supplies was done through his office. Sam would call Miss Alford, Dr. Brooks's secretary, or carry her a list of the items needed. Our supply of X-ray film and printing paper was getting low, so I called Miss Alford and told her what we needed, including some chemicals for developer and fixer solutions. About a week later, Dr. Brooks came into the laboratory and, since I was not in view, asked where I was. Even though I didn't know him, I suspected from the tone of his voice that something was wrong. He came over to where I was working and asked who had told me to order X-ray and photographic supplies. I told him that no one had, but that our supply was so low we needed more. He asked if I didn't know I had to get approval from him or Dr. Blalock. I said I hadn't known that. Then he wanted to know what I was going to do with the supplies and where they were. I took him into the dark room, showed him where they were stored and the box for the printing of pictures. His voice changed, but he left with the parting shot, "I'm not sure I'm not through with you right now." I began thinking about my next job. The same afternoon, Dr. Blalock came into the laboratory and said, "Don't be having run-ins with Dr. Brooks"; he made no further comment.

About a week later, Miss Alford called and said Dr. Brooks wanted to see me in his office. Now I just knew that that was it, that he had decided he was through with me. On the way to his office, I began wondering what condition my carpenter tools were in. I hadn't used any of them for a couple of years. How many had my brother or father borrowed? But when I went into Dr. Brooks's office, I had quite a surprise. Reaching for a stack of X-ray film and notes on one side of his desk, he said, "Come on in, I have something here you have to help me get finished up." He and one of the house officers, Dr. William Raymond, as I recall, were doing some studies on osteomyelitis in the femur, using the legs of rabbits. Dr. Brooks had numerous X rays of which he wanted prints. Also some of the animals were still alive and I was to get X rays of them and make prints of these. Within the next week or so, I had them completed and went over them with him. He found two or three prints too dark and they had to be redone. When I returned the last prints, he was at his desk. He turned toward the window to look at them. Turning back to his desk and barely glancing up at me, he said, "These are all right." Then he resumed work at his desk without further remarks or comments. His manner had completely changed from what it had been the day he had given me the assignment. Was he so engrossed in the paperwork on his desk that he hardly realized he had received the pictures?

This was the total extent of my contact with Dr. Brooks until mid-May 1941. He came into the laboratory then and asked if I was going to Baltimore with Dr. Blalock. I told him I was thinking seriously about it. He said he just wanted me to know that when Dr. Blalock left, there would be no place for me around there, not for me or for Miss Wolff, Dr. Blalock's secretary (who also went to Baltimore). My impression was that he got a good deal of satisfaction out of passing on the information, but he didn't seem to be trying to force my decision in favor of going with Dr. Blalock. Since he never did any research in the laboratory the entire time I was there, I never really had the chance to know him. Occasionally, he would stick his head in the door and ask if Dr. Blalock was there. If he was there, Dr. Brooks would usually stand by the door and Dr. Blalock would go out to talk with him. Weather and time permitting, the two would play golf together, but this was not an every-week event.

During the first two or three years we were at Hopkins, Dr. Blalock had numerous distinguished visitors from all over the country. Most of them were professional friends and colleagues, some just possibly passing through, who stopped by to see how he was doing at his new job as Professor and Chief, and to wish him well. He was proud of his research and it was unusual for him not to bring his visitors to the laboratory. Wondering why I hadn't seen Dr. Brooks, I asked Dr. Blalock why he hadn't been there. Dr. Blalock replied, speaking very seriously: "You know, Vivien, it's strange. Dr. Brooks did everything he possibly could for me to help me get ahead. He liked me when I was a little boy, but since I've grown up, he doesn't like me any more. I can't get him to come." He seemed a little hurt by Dr. Brooks's attitude.

Dr. Blalock's comment gave me some insight into why I had received notice of my termination while he was preparing to leave Vanderbilt. The talk around Vanderbilt had been about Dr. Blalock's going to Hopkins, but Dr. Brooks had asked if I was going to Baltimore with Dr. Blalock. He surely had no intention of closing the laboratory. Again, while giving me notice, Dr. Brooks had also let me know that Frances Wolff would be terminated upon Dr. Blalock's departure. It seemed to me that he wanted to rid himself of anyone and everyone closely associated with Dr. Blalock. No one who might remind him of Alfred Blalock should stay. Certainly Dr. Blalock's secretary and his technician were in this category.

During the summer of 1930, I had not been able to add anything to the money I had saved. I was still hopeful, but in November of that year, The Peoples Bank, the bank in which I had my savings, closed its doors. Even now, it is difficult for me to describe or express my reaction. I knew how to work to earn money; I knew how to save some of that money, so I worked and I saved. Then the bank closes its doors and I can't get the money I worked for and saved. My first feeling was anger—real anger, followed by a mixture of disbelief, resentment, disgust, and hate. Lingering in the background was a loss of trust in everything and everybody. My mind was in a state of utter confusion. I didn't go to work the next day and did not call in. The following morning, when Dr. Blalock asked where I had been, I told him I was sick. He said I must not have been very sick to be back that quickly, and wanted to know what was wrong with me. I told him I had diarrhea. He was upset that I had not even called in.

Even in my frustration, I had to face a sobering reality. Businesses were closing and many factories were slowing production or closing down. Men were walking the streets looking for jobs that did not exist. Things were getting to a point that it seemed to be a matter of survival. For the time being, I felt somewhat secure in that, at least, I had a job. I was out of school for the second year, but I somehow felt that things might change in my favor. I took the whole situation to be an oddity that any day might reverse itself. But it didn't happen. I talked over my situation with Dr. Blalock on several occasions. Once he asked what I could do as a career if I had a bachelor's degree and was unable to go to medical school. I told him that my best chance as of that time would be to teach school. He claimed I could do as well or better financially by staying in the laboratory. He never encouraged me to attempt to continue my education. I don't know if he was aware of the discrepancy that existed in the pay of white and colored teachers, but the shoolteacher's pay situation was to be brought to everyone's attention in the not too distant future.

When Tom Brooks died in 1934, Dr. Harrison hired James E. Lewis to replace him. James and I happened to live in the same neighborhood and James had been a classmate and a fairly close friend of an older brother of mine, so we were not strangers. With Dr. Blalock and Dr. Harrison working on joint projects in 1935 and 1936, James and I were often together. One day, we were discussing how our pay compared to our duties and responsibilities, knowing that on almost any job or position pay was usually determined by job classification. How were we classified? James didn't know and I didn't know. But James did know a secretary who liked to demonstrate how smart and knowledgeable she was. She would tell you almost anything you asked, even confidential information. James knew her quite well and said the first chance he had, he would find out something from her. It took about two weeks or more, but one day he asked her how much one of the white men made. This man was doing about the equivalent of what James and I were doing. Her reply was, "Oh, he's a technician, he makes [so and so much]." There was an appreciable dollar gap between our salaries and his. I told James that he had made the first step, that it was my turn, and that I was going to find out how we were classified. I went to the business manager's office and was told that all of the colored men were classified as janitors. This didn't sound right, for William Gunter, the colored man who worked in the autopsy room, was a licensed embalmer. Assuming that it was at least partially true, James and I wanted to approach our respective bosses with this information then and there, but we knew we would have to plan and use strategy. With Drs. Blalock and Harrison such close friends, we knew that if one was approached, the other would know about it and be on guard. So we decided it would have to be done on a day when we were working with them in our respective laboratories. This meant checking our schedules each day, sometimes even twice a day. At last the day came.

I told Dr. Blalock I had learned that I was classified as a janitor, that for the type of work I was doing, I felt I should be classified as a technician and be put on the pay scale of a technician, which I was pretty sure was higher than janitor pay. He showed a little surprise, saying he didn't know anything about it, but would talk to Miss Alford about it. He also talked to Dr. Harrison about it, for the following morning he asked why I had discussed something like that with James. I told him that people usually discuss mutual problems. Nothing more was ever said about the matter. Several paydays later, both James and I received increases that put our salaries a little more in line with at least one other technician. We never knew or inquired whether we were reclassified or whether they just decided to give us more money to keep us quiet. We were aware that higher classification did not of necessity guarantee us a higher salary but, as individuals, we decided to take the chance, and it produced the desired

results. Had there been an organized complaint by the Negroes performing technical duties, there was a good chance that all kinds of excuses
would have been offered to avoid giving us technician's pay and that lead-
ers of the movement or action would have been summarily fired.

On February 23, 1942, my older brother Harold filed suit on his
own behalf and on behalf of others, challenging the validity of the action
of the Board of Education of Nashville, Tennessee, in establishing fixed
schedules of compensation for teachers which provided considerably
larger salaries for white teachers than for Negro teachers having the same
qualifications.

The case, *Thomas* v. *Hibbits et al.*, was tried in the District Court of
the United States, Nashville Division, without a jury, District Judge Elmer
A. Davies presiding. The Federal Supplement abstracted the case July 28
as follows:

> . . . District Court of the United States had jurisdiction of suit by negro
> teacher challenging validity of action of Board of Education of City of Nash-
> ville in establishing fixed schedules of compensation for teachers which pro-
> vided considerably larger salaries for white teachers than for negro teachers
> having the same qualifications. . . .
>
> . . . The adoption by city Board of Education of separate schedules of
> compensation for white and negro teachers providing for a considerable dif-
> ferential in favor of white teachers based solely on the ground of race and
> color was an unconstitutional "discrimination" violating both the "due pro-
> cess of law" and "equal protection of the law" clauses of the Fourteenth
> Amendment. U.S.C.A. Const. Amend. 14. . . .
>
> Suit by Harold E. Thomas against Louis M. Hibbits and others for a
> declaratory judgment as to the legality of the action of the Board of Educa-
> tion of the City of Nashville in establishing different schedules of compensa-
> tion for white and negro teachers, to recover for services previously rendered
> on the basis of the schedule of compensation established for white teachers,
> and to enjoin future discrimination against negro teachers.
>
> Z. Alexander Looby, of Nashville, Tenn., and Thurgood Marshall, of
> New York City, and Leon Ransom, and William H. Hastie, both of Washing-
> ton, D.C., for plaintiff, Harold E. Thomas.
>
> W. C. Cherry, City Atty. for City of Nashville, E. C. Yokley, Jr., and
> Charles G. Blackard, Asst. City Attys., all of Nashville, Tenn., and Myron
> Evans, of Memphis, Tenn., for defendants.
>
> DAVIES, District Judge.
>
> This cause was tried by the court without a jury, and after hearing all
> the evidence and argument of counsel, the court hereby makes the following
> findings of fact and conclusions of law.
>
> Findings of Fact.
>
> . . . The plaintiff, Harold E. Thomas, is colored, a person of African
> descent and of negro blood. He is a regular teacher in the Pearl Junior High
> School, a public school located in Nashville, Tennessee, and maintained and

operated by the Board of Education of the City of Nashville. He is now completing his sixth year as a teacher in the Public Schools of the City of Nashville, Tennessee, and is paid the sum of $110 per month for his services; this being the amount fixed by the Board of Education for the City of Nashville for negro teachers in their sixth year of teaching experience.

Plaintiff successfully completed the course of instruction provided at Fisk University located at Nashville, Tennessee, which is an accredited college and has been awarded the degree of Master of Sciences from said University. He holds a Collegiate Professional Certificate, which is the highest certificate issued by the Tennessee Board of Education for teaching in public schools at Tennessee, both white and colored. In order to qualify for this certificate, plaintiff met the same requirements as those exacted by the Tennessee Board of Education for all other teachers, white or colored, and he performs the same duties and renders the same services as is required of all other holders of said certificate.

. . . The Pearl Junior High School, where plaintiff teaches, is known as a colored school, all teachers employed therein and all students who attend the school are persons of African descent and of negro blood. It is an integral part of the public school system of the City of Nashville, Tennessee, maintained by and operated under the direction of the Board of Education for the City of Nashville.

. . . The defendants in this cause are the Board of Education of the City of Nashville, all of its members and the Superintendent of Schools for the City of Nashville, Tennessee, who is an administrative officer of the public free school system of Tennessee.

. . . Identical certificates are issued by the State Board of Education to both negro and white teachers.

. . . Among the various duties, prerogatives and official acts of the Board of Education of the City of Nashville, is that of employing and fixing the compensation of the teachers in the public schools of the city. It is required under the Constitution of the State of Tennessee to maintain separate schools for white and colored. For many years the Board of Education has employed its teachers on a fixed salary schedule and has maintained separate salary schedules for white and colored teachers. On September 18, 1940, the Board of Education of the City of Nashville adopted new schedules of salaries for its teachers in the public schools, effective as of September 1st, 1940, and at this time adopted separate schedules for teachers in white schools and in colored schools, which is just another way of saying that it would have a separate schedule for white teachers and colored teachers, inasmuch as only white teachers are employed in the white schools and colored teachers in the colored schools. Under this schedule, a teacher in the Elementary and Junior High Schools, employed in the first year of teaching, is paid $120 per month in the white school, and $95 per month in the colored school; and for the same class of school, a teacher in the fourth year of teaching is paid $135 per month in the white school, and $110 per month in the colored school. Likewise, according to the schedule, a teacher employed for the first year in a senior high school is paid the sum of $140 per month in a white school, and

$100 per month in a colored school; and in the fourth year is paid $170 per month in the white school and $115 per month in the colored school.

. . . The requirements of eligibility for employment as a teacher in the public schools of Nashville, as fixed by the Board of Education relative to experience, qualifications, etc., are the same for colored teachers as for white teachers.

. . . The defendants in their answer state that the discrimination in the amount of salaries paid to white teachers and to colored teachers in favor of the white teachers, is based solely upon the different types of school, that is, colored schools and white schools and does not in any way attempt to make a discrimination in the teachers of the different types of school. This proposition seems to have been more or less abandoned at the trial of the cause where what the defense relied upon was that the differential in the pay of the salaries to the teachers was based solely upon an economic condition in that, colored teachers were more numerous than white teachers, their living conditions less expensive, and that they could be employed to work at a lower salary than white teachers. It is also insisted in the answer filed by the defendant that if the Board of Education should see fit to appoint negro teachers in white schools, their salaries would be based upon the race of their pupils, and not as to the color of the teachers. Granting that this could be true in the abstract, yet it is of considerable import that so far no negro relied upon that the applications from the colored teachers were far more numerous than from white, and that as an economic proposition colored teachers could be secured to work for a smaller salary than white teachers. The court is unable to reconcile these theories with the true facts in the case and therefore finds that the studied and consistent policy of the Board of Education of the City of Nashville is to pay its colored teachers salaries which are considerably lower than the salaries paid to the white teachers, although the eligibility qualifications and experience as required by the Board of Education is the same for both white and colored teachers and that the sole reason for this difference is because of the race and color of the colored teachers.

. . . Plaintiff is entitled, in his own behalf and in behalf of the class whom he represents, to the issuance of an injunction restraining the defendant Board of Education, its officers, agents and employees, from making any discrimination against plaintiff and the class whom he represents in fixing salaries to be paid to school teachers for the next fiscal year and succeeding years on the grounds of race or color.

A decree will be entered accordingly.

Thus, the Board of Education in Nashville, Tennessee, was forced to pay colored teachers by the same salary scale as that set up for white teachers. Many contributors to this court action asked not to be identified for fear of recrimination. Harold (see fig. 8) awaited notice of his assignment for the fall session of school and upon receipt of his notice of assignment resigned from the school system. He also left the teaching profession.

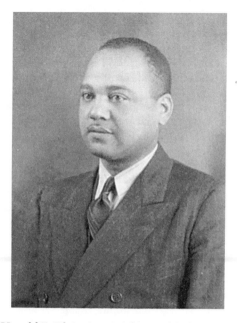

Fig. 8.   In 1942 Harold E. Thomas, a graduate of Fisk University, challenged the validity of the action of the Nashville Board of Education in establishing fixed compensation schedules for teachers, which provided larger salaries for white teachers than for Negro teachers having the same qualifications.

good in report for basics

In the early summer of 1933, I had occasion to be in Macon, Georgia. There I met Clara Beatrice Flanders, a lovely young lady just graduating from high school. I saw her only a few times while there, but she was so appealing that I found myself back in Macon on my vacation in August, having corresponded with her during the interim. We were married on December 22, 1933, and I brought her to Nashville. Our first child, Olga Fay, was born the following year; a second, Theodosia Patricia, was born four years later, in 1938.

A decision had to be made about moving to Baltimore. My wife wanted to leave the full decision to me, but there were a number of factors that we both had to consider. First of all, we had two little girls to take care of, to raise, and to educate. The younger had just turned two, the other was six. Their future would be involved. Next, it was obvious that I liked the type of work in which I was engaged. Since Dr. Brooks had made it clear that I would not be in his laboratory after Dr. Blalock left, and since there was no equivalent laboratory at Vanderbilt or at any other institution in the Nashville area, if I wanted to stay in the field, it meant we would have to move to Baltimore. On the other hand, I could go back into the building trade. By this time, the construction business had sub-

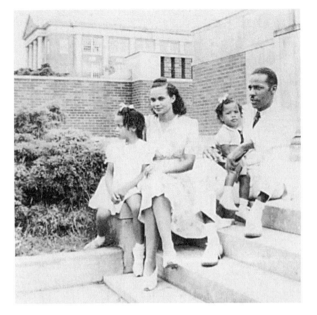

*Vivien Thomas, his wife, Clara, and children
on steps at Tennessee State College in June 1941*

stantially recovered and it would not be too difficult to get back into it. My father and a brother were still in the field. Another factor to be considered was that World War II was raging in Europe and the military draft was in effect in the United States. I was classified 3-A because of dependents. General public feeling was that the United States would almost surely become involved, and I, myself, could not imagine the United States "missing a good war." If we moved to Baltimore and Hopkins, I would be in the employ of a medical school affiliated with a hospital. There was no way of knowing what my draft status would be if and when the country actually became involved in the war, but if I were drafted from Hopkins, I would most likely be placed with a medical unit.

We had never visited Baltimore, nor did we know anyone living there, but we felt that if we moved there and did not like the city and/or its living conditions, or if my working situation was not satisfactory, we could always return to Nashville. Believing that we didn't have much to lose, that we were young and hopefully had many years ahead, we made the decision to move to Baltimore and to Johns Hopkins.

mation all of his choices he debated + how he cared for his children's future. And the drafting.

Part Two

The Hopkins Years

6

Knowing I had never been in Baltimore and knew no one in the city, Dr. Blalock made inquiries of Miss Baker, who had been secretary to Dr. Dean Lewis and was to be one of his secretaries at Hopkins. Thus he suggested that I write to Fred Watson, who was in charge of the animal facilities of Dr. Curt P. Richter, Professor of Psychobiology. I corresponded with Fred, explaining the situation and my plans to move to Baltimore, and he responded with suggestions and welcome advice concerning the move. He also invited me or, rather, suggested that I stay with him and his family for the two or three days it would take to find an apartment. (Fred had his own home in the 1000 block of Harford Road, had not been out looking for an apartment and, therefore, was not aware of the housing shortage that would confront me.)

I arrived in Baltimore on June 20, 1941, several days before Dr. Blalock, who had purchased a house in Guilford. I went to see him the morning after he and his family arrived and told him that I was having difficulty finding satisfactory living quarters. Dr. Blalock invited me to come out and stay with them until I could find a suitable place and I accepted the invitation.

The following morning he asked if I had seen Hopkins and suggested that I accompany him to the hospital so that he could show me around. Having lived in Baltimore during his medical school years, he knew the city well. On the way to the hospital, he pointed out the "Hopkins Dome" from a distance, Harford Road where The Alameda enters Clifton Park as Saint Lo Drive. With the Dome dominating the East Baltimore skyline, the view was very impressive. I had pictured Johns Hopkins as being situated on a beautiful, spacious, tree-lined campus like those of Vanderbilt and Meharry. When we arrived, I was surprised at the close proximity of the buildings within the huge complex and by the Hospital and School of Medicine being so tightly surrounded by row houses. I was, however, very favorably impressed by the appearance of the front of the hospital on Broadway (see fig. 9). Its two curved stone stairways forming an inverted letter U met just across an oval driveway passing at the main entrance. On this landing stood a sundial on a stone pedestal. The stairs were lined on each side with flowers which at that time of year were in full bloom.

Entering under the Dome, my attention was immediately caught by the impressive marble statue of Christ with outstretched hands which

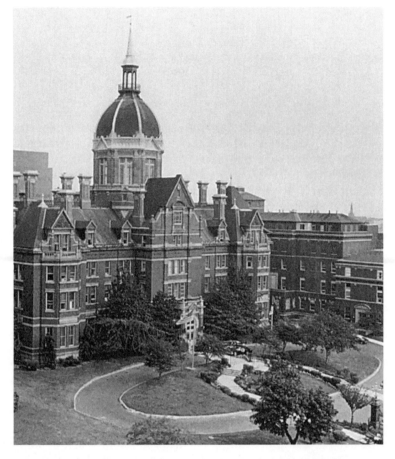

Fig. 9. The Johns Hopkins Hospital with the "Dome," which dominated the east Baltimore skyline. Even though many changes have taken place over the years with the demolition of some of the older buildings and the erection of numerous new ones, this, the Broadway entrance through the administration building, remains the same. Photo courtesy of Johns Hopkins Medical Institutions.

dominates the rotunda. We passed through the rotunda into the "main corridor," which connects all of the buildings in the hospital complex. The corridor was painted the dark green which was the color of the day for hospitals. It had a wooden ceiling from which the paint was peeling. The floor was of smooth-finished concrete. To me it seemed more a tunnel than a corridor. It was not well lighted and was noisy with heavy traffic of patients, staff, and employees. I said to myself, "So this is Hopkins, the great Johns Hopkins, of which I have been hearing as long as I can remember." As we walked, Dr. Blalock told me the names of the buildings we were going by or through and gave the clinical service that occupied each; Marburg, Thayer, the Service building, Brady, and Halsted.

After walking about two city blocks through the corridor, we arrived in the Osler building elevator lobby. This area had a completely different appearance: the walls were buff colored and the floor was of polished marble aggregate. I mentioned this difference in appearance to Dr. Blalock and was told that the building was only about ten years old.

We took the elevator to the fifth floor, his office being on the bridge between Osler and the dispensary (O.P.D.) building. There I met Miss Elizabeth Baker, who remembered Dr. Halsted and had been secretary to Dr. Dean Lewis, Dr. Blalock's predecessor. She was being retained by Dr. Blalock as one of his secretaries. Miss Mable Reese, who had been one of Dr. Halsted's secretaries, was also in the office. That morning, Dr. Blalock stayed in the office only long enough to check a few pieces of mail.

We left the hospital area by way of the Women's Clinic building on Wolfe Street. Across the street was the School of Hygiene and Public Health, with its white stone columns. We headed toward the old Hunterian building most often called the "dog house." It was over a block away and situated behind the impressive white limestone Welch Medical Library. When the Hunterian did come into view, it was obvious that the first part of the name did apply. It was old but so named now because another building constructed later, for the Carnegie Institute of Embryology, was also given the name of John Hunter, the great English surgeon and experimentalist.

Fortunately for me Dr. Blalock had been talking, giving me the history of the anatomy building, the first structure erected on the Medical School grounds, and identifying other buildings as we walked. Even though he had more or less warned me, I was not quite prepared for either the age or odor of the laboratory building. The entrance of the three-story structure was at half level, between lower and middle floors. The building had an impressive appearance, the front being partially vine covered with the laboratories located on the middle and upper levels (see fig. 10). On entering, we were greeted by the odor from the animal quarters below. There was an exhaust system that was supposed to vent the animal odors through ducts directly out through the roof, but it was either inefficient or had been turned off for the day. I learned later that it was inefficient.

We went up the half flight of stairs to the main laboratory floor. Here was the same drab hospital-green paint. Although the outside of the building was of brick, the structure inside was all of wood. In most areas the wood floors were covered with composition tiles. We went into the

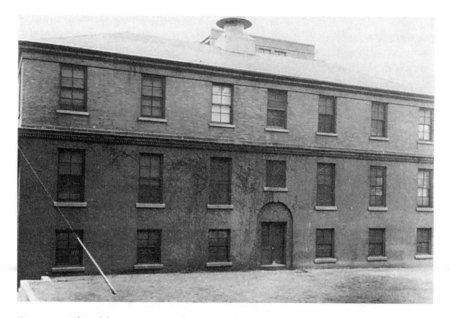

Fig. 10.   The old Hunterian Laboratory, more often called the "dog house," was built in 1905. Much of the medical-surgical history of Johns Hopkins had its origin through research in this building. Dr. William S. Halsted, the first Professor of Surgery, set it up, and Dr. Harvey Cushing oversaw the activity. Photo courtesy of Johns Hopkins Medical Institutions.

general work and classroom area, at the Madison Street end of the building. This large classroom-laboratory area was much like that at Vanderbilt. It was somewhat smaller but accommodated eight animal operating tables. Adjoining it were two smaller rooms, one for the preparation and sterilization of instruments and supplies, the other the scrub room, which also contained the instrument cabinets. I met the laboratory personnel and some of the professional staff. I was then taken to the opposite end of the building where our laboratory and office would be located. Some remodeling had taken place to enlarge the laboratory and to relocate a sink. We discussed the drab appearance of the place and Dr. Blalock asked if I would like to liven it up by painting it before we tried to get down to work. I agreed to paint it if I could change the color. He answered, "Paint it any color you like; you're the one that will be working here." Mr. Burgan (the business manager of the medical school) would get the paint for me.

By this point I would have agreed to almost anything to change what, to me, was a depressing and almost revolting atmosphere. If he had suggested tearing the building down and erecting a new one, I would have gladly accepted the challenge.

The official date for me to begin duty at Hopkins was July 1, 1941. I had arrived in Baltimore on June 20 ahead of my wife and children in order to find housing and to set up for their arrival, but finding a home turned out to be such a difficult and time-consuming effort that, after the guided tour with Dr. Blalock, I did not return to the laboratory until July 7.

Activity in Baltimore was on a full wartime production basis even though the United States was not yet at war. As a center for heavy industry, steel mills, and shipbuilding, and one of the major east coast sea ports, Baltimore was one of the busiest cities in the country. Jobs were plentiful and people were coming from all over the country to fill them. The resulting housing shortage was critical. I contacted rental agencies and drove all over the city and its suburbs looking for an apartment or a house. Many of the apartments that bore "for rent" signs could hardly be classified as fit for human habitation. I finally found an apartment which was really marginal as living quarters, but I decided to take it with the hope of finding something more suitable. I had already decided that, if better living conditions were not shortly forthcoming, we would be back in Nashville before Christmas. Fortunately, we did find a somewhat better place in about two months.

There was quite an adjustment to be made in our mode of living. We had never lived in an apartment, nor were we accustomed to going out the front door directly onto the street, and we had never seen row houses. At that time they were common only to the East Coast. Clara and I had each grown up in areas of the country with individual dwellings with lawns and trees that allowed for some outdoor living—what I called a little elbow room. This type of residence was just about nonexistent, or rather unavailable to Negroes, in the Baltimore area. Moreover the weird and eerie appearance of the city at night puzzled us. We had been in large cities and small towns, but nothing quite matched Baltimore. Was it the influence of Edgar Allen Poe, who had lived here? After a year or so, we finally realized that it was the gas street lights. Baltimore must have been the last major city in the United States to convert its street lighting to electricity. Although we lived in the city for ten years, we never became really accustomed to the congested, treeless, grassless environment. It took us seven or eight years to even consider ourselves permanent residents.

Dr. Blalock had told me that Dr. Edgar J. Poth was the director of the laboratory and that he would get me oriented, give me instruments, and get whatever else in the way of equipment we might need. When I was ready to get started in the laboratory, I went to his office, introduced myself, and related to him what Dr. Blalock had told me. He showed me where instruments and various other supplies and equipment were and said I should make a list of the things I took and a list of any other items we might need. I should not have been, but I was a little surprised in looking over the available equipment and surgical instruments. The regular surgical instruments were in plentiful supply but of an old vintage. Equipment for some of the physiological studies, which were already in the planning stage, was just not available. It reminded me a little of the time I started working with Dr. Blalock at Vanderbilt eleven years earlier, but we had accumulated a tremendous amount of modern equipment in those eleven years. I asked Dr. Poth where I would find Mr. Burgan and told him why I wanted to see him: I had decided on a light gray paint for our laboratory.

During the time I was painting, I was getting our instruments and supplies together and also becoming acquainted with the laboratory personnel. Dr. Blalock had informed me only a week or two after his acceptance of the position that there were no colored people working around Hopkins, but he did not see how this would make any difference or cause any problem. The laboratory staff included Thomas (Tom) Satterfield, the senior technician, a robust, pleasant, businessmantype of individual. In his mid-forties, he was the man in charge, on the ground at all times. He was the equivalent of Sam at Vanderbilt, and he turned out to be my right-hand man.

Adolph Stoll was a little on the heavy side, almost jolly, and always looking for humor in any situation. In his mid-thirties, he knew his job well and was more or less Tom's assistant.

Mrs. Dorman, the stout, elderly maid and housekeeper, spoke with quite an accent, Polish I thought. She also helped with the preparation of linen and sterile supplies.

Ludwig Wolopich, affectionately called Pop, was the animal caretaker. In his early sixties and Austrian born, he spoke fairly good English until something or someone upset him, at which time he would excitedly revert to his native German. When this happened there would be nothing one could do but smile and walk away. He had an assistant or co-worker whose name I can't recall. He left soon after my arrival, and Pop did not want him replaced. Pop invariably had his own way. He was conscientious in caring for the animals, worked endlessly, and the thought of having to replace him was not bearable.

Stuart R. Elliot II was a chemistry technician working with Dr. Poth whose studies were concerned with the effect of the sulfa drugs on the gastrointestinal flora. The poorly absorbed sulfonamides were being evaluated for preoperative preparation of the bowel.

George Elliot, no relation to Stuart, was another chemistry technician with Dr. Poth.

The surgical staff members who had research projects in progress in the laboratory included Dr. Warfield M. Firor, who had been acting chief of surgery for the two years preceding the appointment of Dr. Blalock, Dr. Phillip Price, and Dr. Austin Lamont. They all had private laboratories located on the top (third) floor of the building. With the general situation in the entire institution changing so rapidly, almost abruptly, with the entry of the United States into World War II in December, I did not have the chance to visit their laboratories and become familiar with their research projects.

I took a part of August for vacation, and it was well into September before we were ready to settle down to research. Most of the instruments and supplies needed were readily available and during the elapsed time I had been periodically checking with Dr. Poth about two items that were critical to my getting down to work. The project Dr. Blalock had assigned to me to begin work was to reverse the flow of blood through the mesentery of a segment of small bowel. In the procedure, it would be necessary to dissect the base of the intestinal mesentery in order to expose vessels of adequate size for the anastomoses. The spleen was to be removed and vessels of comparable size in the pedicle used for the anastomoses. With me working alone, exposure in the deep abdomen would be practically impossible without a Balfour retractor. This particular retractor has a third blade, the two major blades giving lateral retraction, the third retracting at one end of the incision.

There were several of the basic retractors in the instrument cabinet and several blades, none of which matched the retractors. A new Balfour retractor was on the list I had submitted to Dr. Poth. I had also requested several spools of 5-o and 6-o Deknatel braided silk and had discussed with him the need for both items. He himself tried to match a blade with a retractor, and he showed me a large spool of fine-twisted silk which he said was used for blood vessel suturing in the laboratory. I explained the difficulty we had encountered with the Johnson and Johnson vascular sutures of twisted silk, but he insisted I try the silk he had. I had taken the liberty of bringing along a supply of J-and-J needles from Vanderbilt, though when I had packed them, I did not know they would be needed so quickly. Dr. Blalock was getting impatient for me to begin. When I relayed this information to Dr. Poth and inquired about the two missing items, he replied that we could not have the Balfour retractor and that I would have to make out with the silk used in the laboratory because they did not use the type I had requested. I did not feel it incumbent upon me to try to force the issue, but I had no alternative but to tell Dr. Blalock what I had been told. The request had surely been in Dr. Poth's hands a sufficient length of time for him either to have consulted with Dr. Blalock about the expenditure if he thought I did not have the authority to make the request or to have told me if there were no funds available.

When I went into Dr. Blalock's office, he was at his desk reading his mail. I related my latest effort to start work and what I had been told by Dr. Poth. His reaction was just about what I had expected. "Who the hell does he think he is? I run this department. Tell him," he broke off, reached for a piece of paper on one side of his desk, and wrote in bold longhand, "Dr. Poth—Get anything Vivien asks for for my work," and signed it "Alfred Blalock." He passed the note to me without even folding it, saying, "Here, give this to him." I had been around Dr. Blalock before and was around him for a long time thereafter, but I never saw him get quite as perturbed as he did on that occasion. Passing the outer office, I had Miss Wolff put the note in an envelope and seal it. I placed the note on the desk in Dr. Poth's office in the laboratory. Normally uncommunicative, he was referred to as "Smiling Eddie" by many members of the surgical staff. The day after the note was left on his desk, I greeted him in the corridor, but my greeting was not acknowledged or returned.

From that day until he left in June the following year, he never spoke to me, even though our offices in the Hunterian were next door to each other. My last two requested items were on my desk one morning about a week later. After that I never made verbal requests, but let him know our needs by written notes placed on his desk. If he wanted or needed additional information about some request I had made, I would find a note on my desk.

When I had everything needed and was ready to begin work, I left a request on his desk for a dog, stating the size and sex, for a given date. When I came in on the specified morning, a note was on my desk giving room and cage number in which I would find the dog. My instruments were already set up so I put them in to sterilize, went to the animal quarters, weighed the dog, and brought him up the steps on a leash. I tied him to the leg of the operating table in my laboratory. Dr. Blalock had suggested that it might be better to confine my work to our laboratory until I could get accustomed to the laboratory scheduling. Although he knew that I would need some help, especially on aseptic procedures, he left me completely on my own to find that help.

Since my relations with the director of the laboratory had so completely deteriorated, I restricted all of the work to our private laboratory until his departure. I went to the work room and asked Tom and Adolph if one of them would assist me in putting the animal to sleep. Tom volunteered. While we were putting the animal to sleep with intravenous Nembutal, Tom asked what time the Professor was coming (everyone referred to Dr. Blalock as "the Professor"). I told him that he was not coming.

Then he asked who was going to do the operation. When I told him that I was, he didn't believe me and said, "Oh, come on now, don't kid me." I told him I wasn't kidding. He stayed around a few minutes, more or less speechless, while I was clipping and shaving the dog and then left. I prepared the skin of the animal and went in to scrub up. After scrubbing, I draped the operative field, put on my gown, and went back to the work room area to have the gown tied and to put on gloves. The scrub room and sterile supplies were at the opposite end of the building.

The laboratory was using what was known as the wet glove technique. Regardless of what the operative schedule was for the day in the laboratory, the first thing Tom did in the morning was to prepare gloves. Two or three pairs of several sizes of gloves would be put in water to boil. While the gloves were boiling, he would flame three or four basins by pouring about an ounce of 95 percent alcohol into each and lighting the alcohol with a match. When the alcohol was burned out, the basins were considered sterile. Bichloride of mercury tablets were then put into each basin and the basins were filled to three-quarters' capacity with water. The gloves that had been boiled were then placed in this solution, with each basin containing a different size glove. Donning the gloves from this solution was relatively easy, but it was virtually impossible to force all the solution from the gloves. As a result, one's hands stayed wet as long as one wore the gloves. This technique was a holdover from the days of Dr. Harvey Cushing, the eminent neurosurgeon who had been in charge of the laboratory in Dr. Halsted's day. It had been used in the general operating rooms of the Hospital and was still being used in the accident room. I did not like the technique and in about two weeks I began preparing my own gloves wrapped dry, with talcum powder, and autoclaving them. On the departure of Dr. Poth, the dry glove technique was adopted for the use of everyone operating in the laboratory.

Not knowing how cooperative people were going to be, I had taken great care to have everything I might need during the operation. Tom and Adolph were busy in other parts of the building, and no one came into the laboratory throughout the procedure. When I had finished I carried the animal back to his cage, cleaned my instruments, and set them up in the tray for next time.

Later that day, Tom came in and asked how I had made out and what the procedure was that I had done. After I gave him a brief description, he said he would like to talk with me a few minutes if I didn't mind and had the time. Our conversation became quite involved. It was mostly a matter of my answering the many questions he asked. Until now the technical staff had assumed that I would be setting up and preparing for the Professor to work, just as they set up and prepared for the other investigators.

What I was doing was something entirely new to them. How long had I been doing this? Did I go to school to learn? How and where did I learn? Who worked with me? Did I usually work alone? We had been talking for about twenty minutes when Tom saw Dr. Poth go into his office. He broke off the conversation, saying he had to go but that we would have to talk some more.

The work went along well for the next two weeks or so with Tom or Adolph giving me about the same amount of help to get started in the mornings and sometimes again in the afternoons. Our conversations started me thinking. Neither Tom nor Adolph had ever heard of a surgical research technician doing what I was doing. Certainly none of the technicians at Hopkins did the work I did. Under the circumstances at least I had the consolation that I was not in competition. Was my position an invention of Dr. Blalock. Was I someone he could teach to do the things he could do and maybe do things he could not do? Surely I was no robot. At what other institution would I be able to find individuals without academic degrees who would fall into my category? Were there others in the laboratories around the country carrying on research in this field as I was doing? I have never known.

Dr. Blalock visited the laboratory two or three times a week. If I was busy, he would often sit at the desk in the adjoining office and look over notes and we would converse through the open doorway. He was extremely busy, but the walk and the visits to the laboratory seemed to relax and refresh him.

In addition to painting the laboratory, I scrubbed, waxed, and buffed the tile floor. As a result, the laboratory actually looked out of place in the old building in which it was located. One day, Dr. Blalock mentioned how filthy the laboratory was getting. Filthy was the right word. Since I was in the laboratory all day, every day, I knew that the place hadn't been cleaned since I started the experimental work. Trash cans hadn't been emptied, the floor under the sink was piled high with used paper towels, the sink hadn't been cleaned, the floor hadn't been swept, the counter tops hadn't been wiped off or dusted. I kept the desk and the small portion of the counter top I used clean, and each day I disposed of operating room waste that might cause odors. Dr. Blalock asked if I couldn't do something about the rest of the laboratory. I told him that I understood Mrs. Dorman was the maid or housekeeper; she was taking care of the rest of the building, right up to our door. Why not our laboratory too? I told him I could clean it but that it would take a whole day to get it back into shape and I was expensive help to be spending my time cleaning. He said, "Good Lord, I hope we aren't getting into trouble already." I answered that we were going to have to face it now or later. I had not cleaned at Vanderbilt and had no intention of cleaning here. There was a short period of complete silence, then he slowly rose from the desk, hesitated a moment and said slowly and deliberately, "All right, you take a day off and get this place cleaned up." He left the laboratory in a brisk walk. From the tone of his voice, I had the feeling that something was going to happen. I spent the next day leisurely cleaning the laboratory and making a thorough job of it. After this, my laboratory and office were always clean when I arrived. I never knew how it was accomplished. There would be no one in the building when I arrived shortly before 8 o'clock each morning. Mrs. Dorman usually came in at 9 o'clock. Since she lived nearby, it was possible that she came in very early to clean the area, then went home and returned at 9 o'clock. There was no noticeable change in the attitude of any of the laboratory personnel. Mrs. Dorman retired for health reasons only months after the departure of Dr. Poth. Knowing Dr. Poth's attitude toward me, I believed he was orchestrating the entire situation. When he left Hopkins, he went to the University of Texas, Galveston campus, as Professor of Surgery, he is still active there as an emeritus professor.

The matter was never mentioned again. When an unpleasant decision had to be made, or any other decision for that matter, Dr. Blalock would follow through and then drop the whole matter from his mind. At least he would never bring it up again unless a follow-up was required. He had more important things to remember.

Telephones in those days were strictly voice telephones with an operator on a switchboard in the hospital and an operator on the switchboard in the Medical School with direct lines between the two. Calls were placed through the operators. From the very beginning, Dr. Blalock invariably placed his calls to me from his inner-office telephone. This was quite upsetting to Miss Baker who evidently was accustomed to placing and receiving all of Dr. Lewis's calls. It also required quite some time for her to become adjusted to my appearing in the office unannounced and without an appointment. It was clearly disconcerting to her not to know if he had called me or if I was there on my own.

At one point after we had been at Hopkins several months, Dr. Blalock telephoned and asked me to bring all of my notes and protocols to his office and bring him up to date on what I had accomplished. I put everything in a manila folder, put on my coat, and headed for the hospital. I entered the hospital through the Womens Clinic. The distance from the Clinic to the Osler building is about a city block along the main corridor. As I passed people, some of them actually stopped in their tracks and stared at me. When I left Dr. Blalock's office, I took a shorter route to the street.

Two or three weeks later I received another call for the same type of update. I put the necessary material in a manila folder, took off my scrub jacket, and put on my shirt, tie, and suit coat. When I arrived at Dr. Blalock's office, he asked why I was dressed like I was. Wasn't I working that day? I told him how I had stopped traffic in the main corridor on my previous visit to his office. I had had a long white coat on. A Negro with a long white coat? Something unseen and unheard of at Hopkins! The way I told it, he was amused and smiled. Fortunately there were no problems in my relations with laboratory personnel, professional staff, or anyone with whom I had to come in direct contact.

Several weeks later I received a telephone call from a reporter for the Afro-American newspaper. He said that he had contacted Dr. Blalock about an interview with me and was told by him that he had nothing to do with it, that it was up to me whether I wanted to grant an interview. Dr. Blalock had given the reporter my telephone number. I told the reporter sure, I would talk to him. He arrived at the appointed time. Passing a few pleasantries, we sat down in the office. He said, "It sure is good to see you here." He wanted to know when I had first come to Hopkins (it was now late November or early December 1941). I told him July 1. What was my job title? Surgical Tecnnician in Research. His third question was "Do they allow you to use the same toilet facilities they use?" If the question had come later in the interview, I might not have reacted as I did. But seeing the direction the so-called interview was taking, I told him that I did not consider my position a racial issue. It was a position that paid a salary. For me, it was a means of a livelihood, as his job was to him. I had been doing the same thing for the past eleven years at Vanderbilt Medical School in Nashville, Tennessee, so to me it was no big deal. I had not even applied for the job. I was asked to fill it because the man thought I could do the job that needed to be done or that he wanted done. I didn't know if Hopkins had a policy about hiring or not hiring Negroes in certain positions or capacities, but if I delivered, they couldn't use me as an excuse to not hire Negroes in any capacity. If he insisted on making a headline story about me being here, they might think about it and form a policy. I told him to just keep me out of his newspaper.

Even though there had been no open hostility or resentment shown toward me, there was no doubt that by the time of this so-called interview, I had become oversensitized to occurrences with racial overtones and was overly conscious of the position in which I found myself. I knew I was something of a curiosity or an oddity around Hopkins. There were constant reminders of race throughout the hospital complex, especially the restrooms along the corridors, which were plainly marked for both race and sex. Most Negro employees wore blue uniforms and were relegated to housekeeping duties. I was ignorant of the general attitude of the Negro community and of its sensitivity about Hopkins.

If the reporter had attempted a real interview by asking questions about the job—exactly what it required of me, how did I get it, how did I get along with the other personnel and employees—or even about my personal affairs or my background, I would have answered his question directly. For those who might wonder what the answer would have been— yes, I was allowed to use the same facilities.

Within a few months after coming to Hopkins, I began to find myself in something of a financial bind. It was and is a pretty well recognized fact that hospitals, schools, and most nonprofit institutions and organizations do not have salary ranges and schedules that are in any way comparable to those in commerce and industry. That Baltimore had become a wartime industrial boomtown only worsened my situation. I explained to Dr. Blalock that I was finding it extremely difficult, almost impossible, to get along on the salary I was receiving, even though it was about 20 percent higher than my salary at Vanderbilt. I had accepted his offer in salary to come to Baltimore in the same good faith I thought he had made it. Probably neither of us had really understood Baltimore's economic situation. His response was to tell me that my salary was more than anyone's in the laboratory and to suggest that I discuss the problem with my wife, that maybe she would have to get a job to help out. I told him that my wife and I had already discussed the matter and that she knew I was going to talk to him. I went on to explain that we had two little girls to be cared for, a fact of which he was already aware. I told him that there were many children on the streets with door keys on strings around their necks but that I intended for my wife to take care of ours, that I thought I had the capability to let her do so except that maybe I had the wrong job. I left his office without waiting for a response. From his tone of voice and from what he had said, I felt that further discussion was useless. My father had done a fairly good job of supplying food, clothing, and shelter, while my mother cared for the five of us. I was fully confident that I could do at least as well and I hoped to do even better for our two children. On his visit to the laboratory the following day, earlier than usual, Dr. Blalock told me that Dr. Dandy had given some money to the department, through the university, with which to increase my salary.

When Dr. Blalock came to Hopkins, he did not have the backing or approval of everyone on the surgical staff. Dr. Walter E. Dandy, the world renowned neurosurgeon, was one of the few on whom he could rely as being 100 percent on his team.

Several years later, Dr. Dandy was planning some work in the laboratory. His son, Walter Jr., who was a medical student, was supposed to have made the arrangements with Tom. But when Dr. Dandy arrived in the operating room area, nothing was set up for him, nor was his son present. He talked to Tom and gave him instructions as to what he wanted to do. While Tom made the necessary preparations, Dr. Dandy walked leisurely back and forth in the hallway. I had never met Dr. Dandy and I was working in my laboratory on the opposite end of the building. When I saw this person dressed in a scrub suit, I asked if I could be of help to him. He smiled saying thanks, he would be all right. Dr. Blalock told me later that he had been quite amused that I hadn't recognized him.

Dr. Dandy's death in April 1946 was a great personal loss to Dr. Blalock. He had been a staunch friend and loyal supporter and Dr. Blalock had always had the utmost respect for him. I learned after his death that he had been very generous in giving financial aid to those in the medical group but no one but the recipient knew of his kind and sympathetic acts.

World War II was already in progress in Europe when we arrived at Hopkins. Everyone was aware of the civilian casualties resulting from the massive bombing raids on London and other large cities in Europe. Thousands of people were buried beneath fallen debris. Medical journals were quick to turn attention to those who survived. Many people who were pinned down by the compression of debris for several hours were in fairly good condition when released from their entrapment. In a few hours their blood pressure would decline and they would go into shock. They would usually respond favorably to treatment. After a period of hours or days, some of these people developed signs of renal damage: urine output diminished and the urine was found to contain albumin and large granular casts. Patients sometimes died in renal failure. The medical profession began to call this sequence of events the Crush Syndrome.

Considering his ever-present interest in the problem of shock, it was natural for Dr. Blalock to begin a series of studies on the Crush Syndrome. He had brought Dr. George W. Duncan from Vanderbilt as part of his team. Duncan was an assistant resident on the surgical house staff, but in the fall of 1941 Dr. Blalock dispatched him to the laboratory. His assignment was to attempt to reproduce, study, and treat the syndrome.

The cases reported in the medical journals were of patients who had had an extremity or a large mass of skeletal muscle crushed. Dr. Blalock decided that we should use one of the posterior extremities as we had in his studies on shock produced by muscle injury. Since the thigh of a dog is almost flat, the femur made it quite difficult to compress or crush the muscle. After numerous changes in design, we were able to develop a device that would crush the muscle without damage to the bone. The pressure exerted by the device also produced ischemia (deficiency of blood supply) of the muscle of the leg.

In the first, or control, series of experiments on shock produced by crushing injuries,[21] the compression device was applied to one of the posterior extremities of dogs which had been anesthetized with Nembutal (30 mg./kg.). The device was left in place for five hours. When it was removed, the leg would swell and there would be a decline in the blood pressure. Blood studies demonstrated a gradual hemoconcentration. Urine examinations revealed some of the granular casts that had been reported clinically. In this control, untreated group, 95 percent of the animals died. It seemed that we had produced a condition in dogs very closely resembling the clinical Crush Syndrome.

Numerous methods of treatment followed. A specially designed and constructed pneumatic cuff or boot was used in the first of these methods. On removal of the compression device, the leg was placed in the boot, and a pressure of forty millimeters of mercury was maintained within the cuff. This pressure, transmitted evenly to the surface of the extremity, reduced the amount of swelling. There was a recovery rate of 75 percent, even though many of the animals showed signs of renal damage, decreased urine output, casts, etc. Several other methods of treatment were investigated including the application of cold and the use of intravenous blood plasma.

We performed a number of studies in an attempt to determine the cause of the shock produced by crushing injuries. In these studies, we attempted to ascertain if toxic products had been produced in the injured tissue during the crush period. Toxemia had been one of the theories advanced as the cause of traumatic shock. To study this, the left thoracic duct was cannulated in the neck. Since most of the lymph flow from all parts of the body enters the venous system at this point, this lymph should contain a large percentage of any toxic products from the injured extremity. The lymph was collected for several hours following the release of the compression of the leg.

To test the lymph for its toxicity, we injected the lymph intravenously into small dogs while monitoring the blood pressure of the recipient. In over half of the recipients, there was a decline in blood pressure, in some a marked decline. Casts were found in the urine in over half of them six hours after the injection. Death occurred subsequently in 25 percent of the recipients.

These findings made it necessary to do a comparison study with lymph obtained from animals in shock produced by simple muscle injury (trauma) as described in the Vanderbilt experiments. In this series, there was a slight decline in blood pressure in only one recipient animal and an actual increase in blood pressure in 90 percent of the dogs. There were no casts found on examination of the urine of the recipients. The different results in these two groups of animals made it seem likely that some toxic substance had been produced in the ischemic extremity during the crush period. No attempt to identify the toxic substance was made.[22]

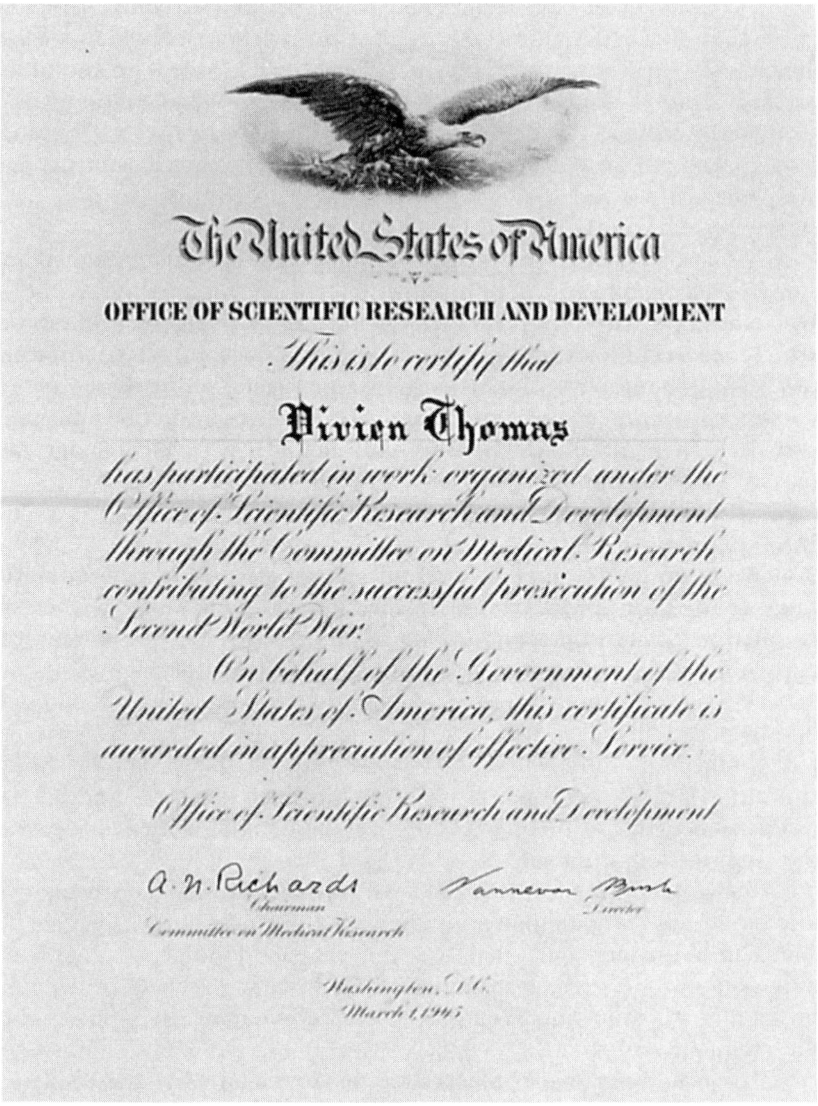

The United States of America

OFFICE OF SCIENTIFIC RESEARCH AND DEVELOPMENT

This is to certify that

Vivien Thomas

has participated in work organized under the Office of Scientific Research and Development through the Committee on Medical Research contributing to the successful prosecution of the Second World War.

On behalf of the Government of the United States of America, this certificate is awarded in appreciation of effective Service.

Office of Scientific Research and Development

A. N. Richards
Chairman
Committee on Medical Research

Vannevar Bush
Director

Washington, D.C.
March 1, 1945

Fig. 11. Certificate of participation in work organized under the Office of Scientific Research and Development through the Committee on Medical Research contributing to the successful prosecution of World War II. The work on shock was deemed essential to the war effort, and my participation in it prevented me from being eligible for the military draft.

The United States had entered the war and with the manpower short-age and restrictions placed on the number of young doctors that could be kept in training, Dr. Blalock had recalled Duncan to the house staff in June 1942.

Dr. Blalock was working in cooperation with the Office of Scientific Research and Development in his studies on shock. As a participant in the project, I was exempt from military service (see fig. 11). My draft sta-tus was 3-A due to dependencies, but every six months I would be re-classified 1-A (eligible to the draft). Each time I received notice of the change in classification, I would give the notice to Dr. Blalock. He, in turn, would fill out the necessary forms and send them to my draft board which was still in Nashville, where I had originally registered. In a few days, I would receive notice of return to my deferment status.

By this time, 95 percent of the medical students were in the armed services, either in the Army Specialized Training Program (ASTP) or the Navy V-12 Program. School was in continuous session throughout the year. Thus the students were completing the normal four-year course in three years, with a group graduating and receiving their M.D. degrees every nine months. A one-week break was given at the end of June and another from Christmas through New Year's Day. That was the full extent of vacation for everyone for the duration of the war.

7

Dr. Blalock approached the problem of coarctation of the aorta after an almost casual mention of the problem by Dr. Edwards A. Park. Several months later Dr. Park was greatly surprised to find a complete manuscript of "The Surgical Treatment of Experimental Coarctation (atresia) of the Aorta"[23] on his desk with himself listed as co-author. He asked to have his name removed, but the Professor would not listen to him.

Coarctation (constriction) of the aorta is a condition that leads to severe hypertension in the head and arms and ultimately death from heart failure or stroke. It is an isolated congenital malformation; that is, it usually does not occur in association with other congenital malformations of the heart and/or great vessels. It is most frequently located just distal to the arch of the aorta at about the level of the ductus ligament, but may occur proximal or distal to this point. The problem was how to get more blood beyond this point of constriction to the lower part of the body and lower extremities. We made numerous attempts to produce a chronic constriction of the aorta. Being unsuccessful in these attempts, Dr. Blalock decided that I should divide the aorta to actually produce atresia and then span the gap in the circulation by using the left subclavian artery (see figs. 12, 13).

In an end-to-end anastomosis, the eversion of the edges of the vessels is accomplished by a relatively simple placement of sutures. By using three stay sutures, triangulating and apposing the ends of the vessels, the operator may rotate the vessels so that any segment of the suture line may be made the anterior segment, and any segment brought into full view. This was the technique we had used in the transplantation of organs and in the divided subclavian artery to divided pulmonary artery anastomoses.

For this end-to-side anastomosis, the vessels could not be rotated, the aorta being in a fixed position. The posterior segment of the anastomosis had to be dealt with *in situ*. It was impossible to visualize the suture from the outside of the vessels due to the fact that the two vessels were running in precisely opposite directions. Placing a continuous everting mattress suture and tightening each stitch as placed was awkward, time consuming, and difficult. I tried taking several stitches before tightening and it worked. Thus, the technique of placing a continuous everting mattress suture loosely across the posterior one-third of the suture line was developed. Putting tension on both ends of the suture material simul-

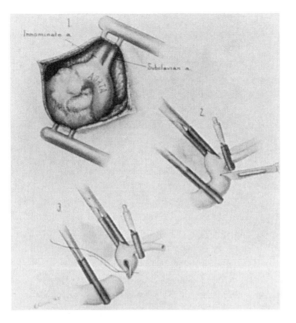

Fig. 12. *Drawings showing steps in creation of experimental coarctation (atresia) of the aorta. 1: Exposure of the aorta and left subclavian artery through an incision in the fourth left intercostal space. 2: Aorta occluded in two places with rubber-shod Allis forceps. The subclavian artery is occluded with a rubber-shod bulldog clamp. It is ligated high in the chest and divided. The aorta is divided. 3: The ends of the aorta are sutured closed. The aortic flow has been permanently interrupted. From Blalock, A., and Park, E. A.: The surgical treatment of experimental co-arctation (atresia) of the aorta, Annals of Surgery 119:445, March 1944, with permission.*

taneously tightened the entire segment of the suture line, thus everting the edges of the vessels. Stay sutures were then placed at each end of this segment of the suture line that had been put in place and the ends of the everting mattress suture anchored to them. Another stay suture was then placed midway of the anterior segment. With slight tension on this third stay suture, the everting mattress suture was then continued, each stitch being tightened as it was placed. This was interrupted midway of the anterior segment by tying it to this third stay suture. On completion of the last third of the suture line, the suture was tied to the first stay suture which was still in place. The occluding clamps were removed from the aorta and the subclavian artery allowing the blood from the subclavian artery to pass into the distal aorta. There was frequently some bleeding from the suture line which could usually be controlled by digital pressure. (I had found much earlier in vascular suturing that light pressure with a gloved

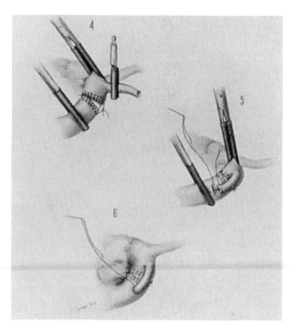

Fig. 13. *The operation for relief of coarctation. 4: A second row of sutures placed for secure closure of ends of aorta. Ends of vessel anchored together to prevent separation. 5: Incision made in side of distal end of aorta. 6: The end of the divided subclavian artery is anastomosed to the opening in the side of the distal aorta. The short, straight threaded needles used for the anastomosis were not available commercially. Longer needles were cut short, and new points honed on them with a fine emery block. This is the type of needle that was used in the first Blue Baby operation. From Blalock, A., and Park, E. A.: The surgical treatment of experimental co-arctation (atresia) of the aorta,* Annals of Surgery 119:445, *March 1944, with permission.*

finger was much more effective in controlling bleeding points than a gauze sponge. The finger could be slid away whereas the gauze sponge would dislodge the clot when it was removed.)

Many of the animals had paralysis of the lower half of the body as a result of the temporary occlusion of the aorta. There was only a 25 percent survival of the animals in good condition after several months. The procedure and the results were published, but the article did not describe the suture technique which I had developed in performing the anastomosis. However, the technique was subsequently described in its use for subclavian pulmonary anastomosis.

Patients with coarctation of the aorta develop varying amounts of collateral circulation, carrying blood around the constriction. These experiments had been performed on animals with no collateral circulation, and it was felt that a patient, having collaterals, would tolerate the procedure without the risk of becoming paraplegic. But it was some time before a patient, whose condition it was thought would be improved by the procedure, was seen in the clinic. During this waiting period, two surgeons, working independently in Europe and in the United States, reported that they had successfully resected coarctations and sutured the ends of the aorta together without resorting to the by-then published subclavian technique, which nevertheless retains its own place as the occasional technical answer in operations for coarctation of the aorta.

Shortly after our arrival at Hopkins, Dr. Blalock had assigned me the problem of the reversal of the blood flow in a segment of small intestine, making no mention of obtaining someone to help me. At that time we barely knew the laboratory technical staff and I had not even seen a medical student. Now again he left me completely on my own as to how to accomplish this coarctation project and to get any assistance or instrumentation that might be needed. As the Professor's good friend and colleague Dr. Tinsley Harrison liked to quote: The three stages of research are (1) The planning, "We need to do . . ."; (2) The work, "You do . . ."; and (3) The report, "I did. . . ."

Bulldog clamps were standard instruments for the temporary occlusion of small blood vessels, but there was no standard instrument for the temporary occlusion of a large vessel such as the aorta. Something had to be found or devised that would occlude the vessel but would not crush and thereby injure it. Looking over instruments in the cabinets, I came upon the Allis forceps. By fitting a length of rubber tubing of proper size and wall thickness over each of the jaws, which do not normally approximate, I was able to get enough pressure between the two jaws to occlude but not injure the aorta. Using a combination of traction and anchor sutures and traction ligatures to get exposure and hold things in place, I proceeded with the series of operations. Sometimes uncut sutures and ligatures used for traction created quite a clutter. Traction was fixed on these uncut ends by anchoring them with hemostats at various locations along the edge of the incision in the chest. After performing the procedure six or eight times one day I had unexpected and top-ranked assistance. Coming into the laboratory and seeing the maze of traction material through which I was working and the struggle I was having, Dr. Blalock said, "Let me help you with that." He asked if I couldn't get a student or someone to help me. Tom was administering anesthesia. Having noticed that the Professor had assisted instead of taking over the procedure, he commented later that I sure did go in for high-powered assistants. Up to this point I had not been given liberty to ask students to assist me. The medical students had helped at Vanderbilt, but with an understanding with Dr. Blalock. Now I was able to get a student to assist on possibly half of these procedures. Their scheduling was rather rigid, leaving them little free time. In this project it was also found that the only available vascular needles, slightly over an inch long, were too awkward and unwieldy to use in an end-to-side anastomosis and had to be shortened.

While Dr. Blalock was considering the use of this bypass procedure in the surgical treatment of coarctation of the aorta in a patient, we discussed an instrument for the occlusion of the aorta. The Allis forcep used on dogs was not large enough for use in the occlusion of the aorta in adult patients. The only instrument in the cabinet which I thought might be modified for the purpose was a long intestinal clamp. This instrument had fine serration of the jaws, but the jaws were too long and so rigid that the aorta might be crushed. I took two of them to Jones in the machine shop to have them modified. The jaws were shortened to four inches, half the original length, a guide pin was put in one jaw of each clamp near the tip to keep the jaws in alignment, and a slot was machined longitudinally into each jaw. These slots served a dual purpose: they diminished the jaws' rigidity and thereby rendered them slightly flexible and, along with the fine serrations, they reduced the risk of slipping. The instrument was standard in the operating room at Johns Hopkins for years until supplanted by the much later developed Pott's instrument. The instrument is currently listed in surgical instrument catalogues (Sklar) as the Johns Hopkins coarctation clamp (see fig. 14).

It was during this same time period that Dr. Mark Ravitch, the surgical resident, came into the laboratory with an ordinary paper stapler he

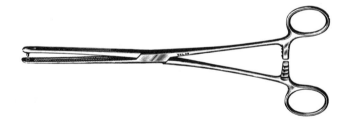

Fig. 14. This coarctation clamp, used clinically for the occlusion of the aorta in the surgical treatment of coarctation of the aorta, was an intestinal clamp that I had modified by reducing the length of the jaws, placing a guide pin near the tip and machining slots the length of the jaws, reducing the rigidity and thereby preventing crushing of the vessel. The slots or grooves also reduced the risk of the aorta's slipping from the instrument. It is listed in the J. Sklar instrument catalog as the Johns Hopkins Coarctation Clamp. Courtesy of J. Sklar Manufacturing Company, Inc., New York.

had picked up from his desk. He had read that Dr. Lahey was using a von Petz stapling machine in performing gastrectomies and was so impressed by the idea that he asked Dr. Blalock for such a stapler. Peeved at being told that it was too expensive, he had his paper stapler sterilized so that he could try it on the bowel of a dog. Of course, the slamming and banging of the stapler literally smashed the bowel and the sterilization (the stapler was boiled in a fish kettle) dissolved the adhesive that held the staples together allowing them to feed too easily. It had been a heroic try but a dismal failure. If he had taken the time it might have been possible to modify the stapler for his purpose. As was true in this case, too often we give up on some idea only to see, in the literature at a later date, that someone else has developed it.

Even though he was back on the house staff, Duncan was working on a joint civilian shock project with Stanley J. Sarnoff, a Fellow in Surgery, and C. Martin Rhode.[24] The latter was on the house staff of the University of Maryland Hospital. This project was done under a contract recommended by the Committee on Medical Research between the Office of Scientific Research and Development and the Johns Hopkins University. A chemistry technician was needed and Duncan was able to secure the services of Clara Belle Puryear, whom he had known at Vanderbilt.

On the termination of this project, Clara Belle began working with us in the Hunterian Laboratory. Duncan also found the time to carry out some additional studies on the shock problem on which she worked.[25] Ultimately, both Duncan and Rhode were called into the armed forces. After the war, Clara Belle and Dr. Rhode were married and they later moved to the Veterans Administration Hospital in Augusta, Georgia, where he had been named Chief of Surgical Services.

Before beginning studies on the utilization of oxygen by the brain in traumatic shock, Dr. Blalock and I had our usual informal discussions about the project, methods of producing shock, observations to be taken, and a broad general outline of the experiments to be performed. After we came to Hopkins, Dr. Blalock always kept in close touch but never tried to set down a rigid protocol for experiments or work out a day-to-day work schedule. His administrative, teaching, and clinical duties left little time for much else. His visits to the laboratory were sometimes restricted to once or twice a week and some of these visits were for only five or ten minutes.

Samples of the cerebral venous blood were to be obtained from the confluence of the venous sinuses (torcular Herophili) which lies beneath the skull at its base posteriorly. I had had a small metal cannula made, tapered and threaded at one end. This cannula was screwed into a small hole drilled into the skull. The taper of the cannula insured a snug fit. An 18 g. spinal needle was slip fitted in the lumen of the cannula and it was only necessary to remove the obturator from the needle and connect a syringe whenever a venous blood specimen was needed. Jones in the machine shop had made it up for us.

The length of time required to produce traumatic shock is so unpredictable that the experiments were between eight and fourteen hours in duration. This being true, I set up for the experiments to be performed on a Monday, Wednesday, Friday basis. Dr. Blalock was aware of the general progress of the project by his periodic visits to the laboratory, but he happened into the laboratory on one of the off days (Tuesday or Thursday). He inquired of Tom where I was. He was told that we had worked late the night before and were taking a day off. It was not unusual for us to get out of the laboratory as late as midnight, after having taken a break from 6 to 7 o'clock. What I was actually doing was to come in for two or three hours on the alternate afternoons to check the notes, calculations, and tabulations from the previous day's experiment to be sure everything was up-to-date. This was the way he was usually given results. I would also get the laboratory in order and set up for the next day's experiment. The next morning, Dr. Blalock met me at the laboratory at about 7:30 (I always tried to get started by 8 a.m. even though our official hours were 9 a.m. to 5 p.m.). He asked about the day before, so I went into detail about what we were doing and the reason for the schedule. I told him that in studying shock, my impression was still that it was preferable to get observations over a longer period of time after shock was produced as we had done for years rather than try to confine the entire experiment to a seven- or eight-hour day. He was quite upset and stomped out saying that even if we worked a few hours overtime, it was no excuse for not getting something done every day.

Clara Belle came in about 9 a.m. and I told her what had transpired and that we weren't doing any more of the experiments on shock until he set up a protocol. We went ahead with some other surgical research projects which had been sidelined for the time being. It was over a week before he came back on his rounds. I brought him up-to-date on what we were doing. He asked how many of the experiments we had done on the sinus project. When I told him we had not done any and that I didn't know what he wanted, I thought he would go through the roof. He was furious. I knew there was no point in trying to talk to him, so I made no attempt to. He was away for about another week. When he returned, I was in the office writing up notes on the other work in progress. As was usual, I got up when he came in. His first question was how many of the sinus experiments we had done. I told him pretty flatly that we had not done any and that he was going to have to decide whether he wanted the series completed with eight-hour experiments or with the longer version, which I felt we would get more out of. He turned and slowly walked away, saying in a normal voice, "Vivien, you do them however you want to. I just want them done." We went ahead with the protocol as I had set it up.

At Vanderbilt Dr. Blalock and I, or a Fellow and I, had alternated on observations and/or determinations to be made late at night or worked straight through the evening if necessary to complete an experiment. Duncan and I had done the same on the Crush Syndrome studies about two years earlier. For these present studies, I was, from a practical viewpoint, carrying the full load so that if an experiment was in progress, I was the responsible person even though Clara Belle was working with me. Dr. Blalock never gave me the time or chance to call to his attention the difference in these circumstances.

Dr. Alan C. Woods, Jr., has been quoted as saying, "It was extremely difficult to tell if Dr. Blalock had the original idea for a particular technique or if it was Vivien Thomas, they worked so smoothly together." [27] During these studies on shock, no one would have suspected that there was anything unpleasant going on between us. His periodic visits were made and progress reports given. He would make his comments, ask questions, and make suggestions. I use the word *suggestions* because I always felt that whatever he said during such sessions was open to discussion and/or even countersuggestion. Dr. Blalock said things in a manner that would stimulate discussion and sometimes, if no comment was forthcoming, would ask flatly what I thought. My general impression was that he wanted all the ideas and opinions available in any given instance or on any subject. He would usually listen closely to other points of view, weigh them, and make the final decision. This was the only time he allowed a project to become stalled after it was underway. This was also the most difficult experience we ever had in achieving an understanding.

Had Clara Belle not been working with us on the project, she would never have known what was going on. But knowing was almost too much for her. She sweated it out, but it made her quite nervous. When the project was completed, we had studied shock produced by hemorrhage, trauma, burns, and by the use of tourniquets. At the end of Dr. Blalock's published report of the studies, in the "fine print," he states "Clara Belle Puryear and Vivien Thomas rendered valuable technical aid." [26] We had.

At Vanderbilt Dr. Blalock had had an office in the laboratory area. Until the last year or so, all notes, protocols, and records were kept in folders on his desk, being placed there at the completion of each day's work. There he would work on them in late afternoon or evening or carry

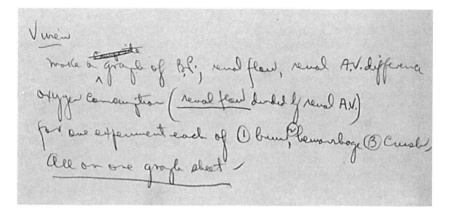

Fig. 15.   A note from Dr. Blalock. While I was busy elsewhere, the Professor went over data on his experiments. After he left, I found the above note, which refers to the effect on the completely denervated (transplanted to neck) kidney of shock produced by the methods mentioned here. The work was never published.

them home with him. In this way he took care of all the paper work. His main office was located on the same floor in the connecting corridor. At Johns Hopkins, the situation was much different with his office being located two or more blocks from the laboratory. His visits to the laboratory were periodic and limited in frequency and the time spent on each visit. Under these circumstances, even though he had not asked that it be done, I tried to keep records and notes condensed and tabulated in a manner that would require the least amount of his time to follow the progress of the various research projects. Even with the notes, calculations, the organization of data, and the tabulation of the results of his experimental work in the laboratory, he would still ask for a little more (see fig. 15). If no Fellow was working with us at or near the end of a project, Dr. Blalock would take the entire folder with him. If more work was needed on the project, he would return the folder and outline the additional experiments required. Inasmuch as he was able to spend only limited time in the laboratory to observe experiments, he was almost completely dependent upon my notes. Over the Hopkins years, it was not uncommon for him to call me while writing a paper. On these calls he would say something like, "Vivien, I want you to listen to this." He would then proceed to read two or three sentences from his manuscript and then ask, "Is that your impression?" On other occasions he might say, "On such and such experiments, can I say so and so?" or "Is it all right if I say so and so?" These notes and records of his experiments would be filed in Dr. Blalock's office.

When a Fellow or others were working on the team, they would usually take possession of the notes and records and these would become part of their file. Very few of these notes and records remained in the laboratory file. In the main, the material left in the file consisted of data and protocols of incomplete, unpublished studies and records of experiments not included in reports of projects. Other records left were reports, some of which I had co-authored.

8

One morning in 1943, Dr. Blalock called to ask what I was doing and if I would be free by late morning. He said a Dr. Taussig had a problem she wanted to discuss and that they should meet in the laboratory so that I could be in on the discussion. He arrived about ten minutes before the appointed time; we talked about the progress of current projects, but the upcoming discussion was not mentioned.

When Dr. Taussig arrived Dr. Blalock introduced us. I had not met her, since she was headquartered in the Hospital and I, in the laboratory. I was to learn later that Dr. Helen B. Taussig was the Director of the Cardiac Clinic in the Harriet Lane Home for Invalid Children at the Hospital. She was a pediatric cardiologist, a skillful diagnostician and an outstanding authority on congenital heart disease.

Dr. Blalock restated what he had said on the telephone and turned to her. She was tall and slender with a pleasant personality and spoke with a distinct New England accent. I don't know how much discussion they had held previously, but she went into great detail about the problems of patients with cyanotic heart disease. There were other types, but she said she was particularly interested in the tetralogy of Fallot (Blue Baby). She described to us the anatomical abnormalities of the heart—the interventricular septal defect, the stenosis (constriction) of the pulmonary artery, how the aorta overrode the septum and the hypertrophy of the right ventricle. She explained the mechanism of how in the presence of the stenosis of the pulmonary artery a varying amount of venous blood was shunted through the defect in the septum out through the aorta into the general circulation and how the amount of the shunting was compounded by the aorta's overriding (straddling) the septal defect. Thus she explained that, under these conditions, there was not sufficient blood getting through to the lungs to be oxygenated.

She also told us of the physical findings, describing the clubbing of the fingers and toes, the blue appearance of the mucous membranes and nail beds, the lack of tolerance to exercise, and the tendency of afflicted children to squat to rest. She told us that they almost invariably had polycythemia (an increased number of red blood cells). She said she had followed these patients in the clinic and seen their condition gradually deteriorate until they finally succumbed, there being no known medical help for them. She expressed her belief that, by surgical means, it should be possible to do something to get more blood to the lungs, as a plumber

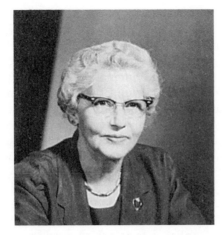

Helen B. Taussig, M.D., c. 1965

changes pipes around, but gave us no hint as to how this could be accomplished—what pipes to put where. She left us with the problem. She had been very sincere in her presentation and had expressed her deep concern about the plight of these patients. I personally had no further contact or communication with her until the project was completed and I began to work with her and her patients in the cardiac clinic.

Dr. Taussig had accumulated a sizable collection of these congenitally defective hearts in the museum in the Pathology building. I spent hours and days poring over, examining and studying these preserved specimens trying to figure out if and how it would ever be possible to create such a model to study and to attempt surgical treatment. If Dr. Taussig had witnessed the autopsy and examined these numerous hearts, each representing a former patient, one could well appreciate her feeling of utter helplessness. She had given a good verbal description of the abnormalities that existed in the hearts of these patients with congenital cyanotic heart disease. I had never seen or examined a defective heart, and what I actually saw defies verbal description except in highly technical terms. I was amazed that some of these patients had survived as long as they had, or had survived at all in view of the defective condition of their hearts. While attempting procedures on an earlier project that had been particularly difficult, I had asked the Professor why he didn't find some easier project. He replied that all the easy things had been done. The reproduction of any of the conditions that existed in these congenitally defective hearts would surely not be easy. Yet, to test any curative operation we first had to reproduce the condition in an experimental animal.

During this period, shock as produced by crush injuries was still being investigated. Dr. Blalock eventually brought up the subject of our session with Dr. Taussig and asked what I thought of the problem and how we could best approach it. I told him I had examined a great number of hearts in the museum and that the only part of the condition I thought we could possibly reproduce was pulmonary stenosis, the other conditions being too complicated to attempt. It was never mentioned during this discussion or at the session with Dr. Taussig, but I am sure both of us were aware of what operative procedure was to be tested if and when we were able to produce a model on which to test it. In attempts to produce pulmonary hypertension at Vanderbilt in 1938, a systemic vessel—the subclavian artery—had been anastomosed to the pulmonary artery. The procedure did not produce the hoped-for theoretical results in normal animals, which we had wanted to study. That is, the blood under systemic pressure, when shunted into the pulmonary artery, did not raise the pressure in the pulmonary circulation as we had theorized. Our task was to produce a model of cardiac defects, which would produce cyanosis that we could attempt to treat.*

Dogs and most other domestic animals, unlike humans, do not have a fixed mediastinum dividing the right and left sides of the chest. In dogs the thin, delicate, transparent membrane that partitions the two sides of the chest allows both lungs to collapse if one side of the chest is opened. Therefore, in laboratory animals an intratracheal catheter is required to administer anesthesia to achieve positive pressure in the lungs. This method was in use in the laboratory at Vanderbilt when I began working there in 1930. Complete collapse does not occur in humans who, with a relatively fixed mediastinum, have some function in the lung on the opposite side if one side of the chest is opened. Many hospitals were administering intratracheal anesthesia in patients, but in 1943 the technique was not yet being used at Johns Hopkins. (As stated in the first Blalock-Taussig paper,[28] open anesthesia was used in the first Blue Baby operations. Intratracheal tubes were used later.)

There was no apparatus or equipment available in the laboratory for administering positive-pressure anesthesia to experimental animals. Because cost was a prime factor, a clinical machine could not be considered. In the illustrated apparatus (see figs. 16, 17), the ether reservoir had been devised by someone in the laboratory long before my arrival. With a stream of compressed air flowing through the ether reservoir, and from it, to a tube inserted in the trachea, positive-pressure respirations were produced by intermittently compressing the trachea around the tube in the trachea to inflate the lungs, then releasing the compression to allow them to deflate. This was repeated ten to sixteen times per minute for as long as was necessary to keep the chest open, sometimes for an hour or

---

*Keep in mind that in 1943 this problem could not be approached with "arm chair strategy." There was no literature on attempts to solve the problem. To the author's knowledge, these were the first attempts, and many were of necessity by trial and error. To repeat Dr. Taussig's statement, "There was no known medical help for them [the patients with congenital cyanotic heart disease]."

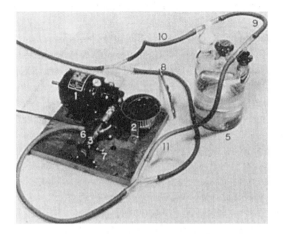

Fig. 16.   An apparatus for anesthesia in experimental thoracic surgery. Necessity being the mother of invention, this apparatus was devised on the urging of Tom Satterfield, who complained of the wear and tear on his hands from manually giving positive-pressure anesthesia. This, the original apparatus, had been in use for over six years when a description appeared in Surgery in June 1950. Photograph of the apparatus shows motor (1), rheostat (2), interrupting valve (3), connected to motor by means of a flexible coupling (4). Air or oxygen is blown over ether in Woulff bottle (5) to enter valve (6) and emerge from nipple (7) to enter tubing leading to an endotracheal catheter. Concentration of ether vapor may be regulated by clamps at any combination of one or two points (8), (9), or (10). During expiration, the gases are exhaled through an exhaust opening in valve, marked by arrow. From Hanlon, C. R.; Johns, T. N. P.; and Thomas, V.: An apparatus for anesthesia in experimental thoracic surgery, Journal of Thoracic Surgery 19(6): 887, June 1950, with permission.

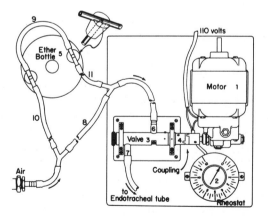

Fig. 17.   Diagram of apparatus for anesthesia in experimental thoracic surgery. The numbers in photograph (fig. 16) and diagram correspond. From Hanlon, C. R.; Johns, T. N. P.; and Thomas, V.: An apparatus for anesthesia in experimental thoracic surgery, Journal of Thoracic Surgery 19(6): 887, June 1950, with permission.

more. This was Tom Satterfield's assignment in experiments in which it was necessary to open the chest. I had done the series of about forty experiments on the coarctation project using this technique. The project had been carried out over a period of several months, as it was being done concurrently with continuing shock studies.

Tom had not complained, but when he saw that I was beginning a new series of operations, he immediately began to complain that compressing the trachea was wearing his hands out. I told him of the effort I was making to procure an apparatus like the one we had used at Vanderbilt. This apparatus had operated on the principle of the windshield wiper, to interrupt intermittently the flow of air to the lungs. Several weeks passed and he inquired as to what progress I was making in getting one. When I told him I was having no success, he wouldn't accept that as an excuse, saying that if I couldn't get one, I was smart enough to make one and should get busy because his hands were going fast. I knew him well enough to know that he was serious, even though he was talking in a half-joking manner. It didn't take much imagination to appreciate what he was saying about his hands, so I didn't waste time.

Working with William O. Jones, the Medical School machinist, we designed a simple motor-driven valve that would intermittently interrupt the flow of air to the lungs and allow time for the lungs to deflate. The ratio of time on (inflation) to time off (deflation) was worked out, essentially by trial and error. The apparatus, although a long way from being physiologically perfect, served our purpose well; it was standard in the Hunterian Laboratory for years and was supplied by me to surgical investigators who had worked at Hopkins and wanted the same simple and dependable apparatus now that they had set up laboratories of their own elsewhere.[29] In order to obtain positive-pressure anesthesia with the apparatus, it was necessary to have a seal between the endotracheal tube and the trachea itself; thus an inflatable cuff was used on the tube. These double-walled cuffs are made of a thin rubber tubing (penrose drain) and are available commercially. In the laboratory, we found that the clinical models of endotracheal tubes with cuffs were not as substantial as might be desired. I had Jones make endotracheal tubes of polished brass in two sizes (3/8- and 1/2-inch diameter), with grooves near the end for tying on penrose drain and a small inner (1/16-inch diameter) tubing through which the penrose drain could be inflated. Only slight curvature of the endotracheal tube is necessary because the jaws and trachea of a dog are almost on a straight line. These tubes were much more economical, since only the penrose drain had to be replaced if an air leak occurred, and the brass endotracheal tube lasted forever (see fig. 18).

The experimental surgical procedures for Blue Baby research were performed on dogs. Anatomically, the heart and the arrangement of the great vessels are much like those of the human. The sizes of the vessels are comparable to those of an infant or a small child. The operations were

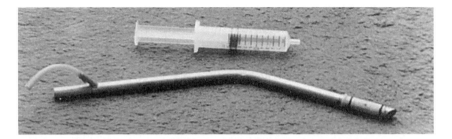

Fig. 18. *Endotracheal catheter made of polished brass tubing in ⅜- and ½-inch diameters. The brass tube, with Penrose tubing tied on with silk serving as a balloon (right end), was more substantial and economical for laboratory use than commercial models. The balloon is inflated with a syringe connected to side arm at left through a very small indwelling tube. If an air leak develops, only the Penrose tubing must be replaced.*

performed using aseptic surgical techniques. A premedication of morphine sulfate and atropine sulfate was given to all of the experimental animals, and positive-pressure ether anesthesia was used.

Dr. Blalock and I agreed on attempting to constrict the pulmonary artery by tying heavy linen ligature material around it. Nothing whatever happened in these animals despite the fact that the ligatures had been tied down to constrict the vessel to the limit of the heart's acute tolerance. When the animals were eventually sacrificed and autopsied, it was found that the ligatures had cut through the wall of the pulmonary artery, one segment of the encircling ligature lying across the lumen of the vessel— just as wire will gradually cut through ice, and water refreeze behind the cut.

Next, we tested a series of animals in which umbilical tape was used to constrict the vessel, the idea being that the tape was broad and less likely to cut through. The results were the same as with the linen ligature. Segments of rubber tubing of the desired caliber were slit and sutured around the pulmonary artery. These segments of tubing eroded the vessel; thus the animals usually died of hemorrhage, as did those in a series in which a band of ox fascia was used. A large silver clamp (Goldblatt clamp) would either erode the vessel if applied loosely or not be tolerated if too much constriction of the pulmonary artery was produced.

In the previous two years, we had concentrated on shock, due to the war and the problems it presented. The coarctation project, however, had been "wedged in," so to speak. Dr. Blalock had not shown the interest in the Blue Baby that one might have expected, possibly because of more pressing problems.

Since we were completing a series of studies on shock, more time could be devoted to the study of Blue Babies. Thus we discussed the overall problem at length and reviewed the results of our attempts to produce pulmonary stenosis.

We had been determining the arterial saturations on the experimental animals, all with negative results. With a little more thought and attention given to these experiments, which had begun as a secondary project, we would have realized that it would be impossible to produce an unsaturation of the arterial blood in the general circulation without some type of shunt. That is, to reduce the amount of blood passing through the lungs for oxygenation would also reduce the quantity of blood circulating through the systemic arteries. This blood would be fully oxygenated unless there was a shunt by which some unoxygenated venous blood returning from the body bypassed the lungs and went out to the body through the aorta.

During one of our discussions, Dr. Blalock presented the idea of producing pulmonary arteriovenous fistulae. This procedure would produce arterial blood unsaturation by shunting some of the unoxygenated right heart blood directly to the left side of the heart without passing through the lung. The pulmonary artery and vein on the right side lie in close proximity and are parallel, so I began by making a fistula between them. This was accomplished by dissecting and isolating a segment of each vessel between bulldog clamps. A longitudinal incision about one centimeter long was made in these isolated segments on the facing side of each vessel. The edge of the incision in the pulmonary artery was then sutured to the matching edge of the pulmonary vein; that is, instead of closing the incision in each vessel, the edge of the incision in one vessel was sutured to the matching edge of the incision in the opposite vessel. Thus an opening or fistula was produced between the two vessels (see fig. 19A). This procedure, which was carried out on several animals, produced the desired unsaturation, but all the animals died in one to three days with hemorrhagic congestion of the right lung due to the venous back pressure.

In order to avoid this complication, we discussed the possibility of making a smaller fistula, but Dr. Blalock decided that I should remove the entire lung on the right side and suture the proximal ends of the right pulmonary artery and the superior pulmonary vein together (see fig. 19B). In this way, no lung tissue would remain distal to a fistula, and the blood being pumped from the right side of the heart toward the right lung would return to the left side of the heart without being oxygenated. The dogs in these experiments all became cyanotic and had little tolerance to exercise. They developed polycythemia with an almost 50 percent increase in red blood count and hematocrit (packed red-cell volume). The oxygen saturation of the arterial blood declined about 25 percent, from 95 percent to 70–75 percent. The picture presented by these results was not as severe as that often seen in patients, but this was the type of blood-analysis picture we were attempting to produce.

Unfortunately, the preparation would not allow us to perform a sub-

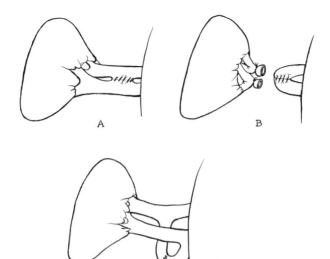

Fig. 19. Pulmonary arteriovenous fistula. These sketches illustrate types of pulmonary arteriovenous shunts used in attempts to produce arterial oxygen unsaturation or cyanosis. The pulmonary artery is shown superiorly on the right side of the chest in each. A: Side-to-side anastomosis of the pulmonary artery and vein of the cardiac and apical lobes of lung; the lobes of lung are left intact. B: Apical and cardiac lobes of lung removed and an anastomosis performed between proximal ends of the pulmonary artery and vein. C: Diaphragmatic and intermediate lobes of lung removed and an anastomosis performed between the proximal ends of the pulmonary artery and vein. This procedure, combined with the removal of the diaphragmatic lobe of lung on the left without the creation of a fistula, produced an arterial oxygen unsaturation in which the effect of the creation of an artificial ductus arteriosus could be determined.

clavian artery to pulmonary artery anastomosis. To accomplish this, it would be necessary to occlude the pulmonary artery to the remaining lung. We had already removed the entire right lung; thus the dogs would not tolerate occlusion of the single, left pulmonary artery during performance of the corrective operation we proposed. However, we had established that the principle of the pulmonary arteriovenous fistula would produce the desired oxygen unsaturation. We decided to remove individual lobes of lung and suture together the proximal ends of the artery and vein of each lobe. In this manner, a portion of lung tissue could be removed from each side of the chest, thereby allowing occlusion of either right or left main pulmonary artery during the creation of a subclavian-artery-to-pulmonary-artery shunt.

Dogs have four lobes of lung on the right side of the chest and three lobes on the left side. On the right side, the branches of the artery and vein of the diaphragmatic and intermediate lobes form single trunks. These two lobes were removed, and the proximal ends of the single artery and vein of the two excised lobes were anastomosed (see fig. 19C). The size and position of the vessels allowed the production of a widely patent fistula.

This part of the procedure was well tolerated. The percentage of oxygen saturation of the arterial blood declined, but although lower than normal in all the animals, in most instances it was not as low as desired. A second fistula was produced after resection of the diaphragmatic lobe of the left lung, but many of the animals died during or after this second procedure. In several animals, the left lower lobe was resected without the creation of a fistula, thereby reducing the amount of effective lung tissue for oxygenation of the blood and forcing more blood to pass through the fistula already produced on the right side.

Very low percentages of arterial oxygen saturation had been produced in some animals, but all had died during subsequent attempts to perform the subclavian-artery-to-pulmonary-artery anastomosis. In view of this, it became quite obvious that the testing of the effect of creating such an anastomosis could not be carried out on animals in which such low and critical arterial oxygen saturations had been produced.

The procedure that had been performed in the experiments at Vanderbilt in attempts to produce pulmonary hypertension had been accomplished by dividing the left pulmonary artery and anastomosing the proximal end of the divided subclavian artery to the distal end of the divided pulmonary artery. This procedure isolated the left lung and circulated only systemic arterial blood through it. The better procedure for our present purposes seemed to be to leave the entire pulmonary circulation intact, thus allowing the increased blood flow to be distributed to both lungs. This required anastomosing the end of the divided subclavian artery to the side of the pulmonary artery, which would produce a blood-flow effect like that in patent ductus arteriosus, thus an artificial ductus arteriosus.

It turned out that the production of an artificial ductus in animals with a less-severe degree of oxygen unsaturation was tolerated. There was a significant increase in the percentage of oxygen saturation of the arterial blood in most instances, the results being fair in the remainder.[30]

For the production of the artificial ductus arteriosus, an incision was made through the left fourth-intercostal space. The left subclavian artery was exposed and dissected free for its entire length; then it was ligated as high as possible in the chest. After a bulldog clamp was placed on it at its base close to the aorta, the vessel was divided just proximal to the ligature. The left pulmonary artery was dissected free, and a length of umbilical tape passed beneath it. A segment of the pulmonary artery was isolated between bulldog clamps and cleaned of adventitia. Moderate traction was put on the umbilical tape that held the vessel in place for the anastomosis. A transverse incision was made in the isolated segment of the pulmonary artery. The incision was made a little longer than would be required to accommodate the circumference of the free end of the divided subclavian artery. This was to assure that the suture line was not smaller or shorter than the end of the subclavian artery, thus constricting the suture line. This free end of the artery was then sutured into the opening in the pulmonary artery.

The technique of performing the end-to-side anastomosis of vessels had actually been developed in studies on the surgical treatment of experimental coarctation of the aorta, which have been discussed previously.

In producing a model in which to attempt surgical treatment of the abnormality, the amount of blood reaching the lungs for oxygenation had been decreased by shunting a portion of it away, as happens in the tetralogy. In the reproduction of the problem in tetralogy patients, by substituting a pulmonary arteriovenous fistula for the interventricular septal defect the circulation had been so altered that mixed arterial and venous blood entered the systemic circulation. Thus, two of the basic conditions had been duplicated: (1) reduced percentage flow of systemic blood through the lung and (2) a mixture of arterial and venous blood flowing in the systemic circulation. This was not an exact replica of the abnormalities, but at least some of the clinical findings had been produced. The procedure had produced a reduced arterial oxygen saturation, cyanosis, and polycythemia.

In the surgical treatment of the model, an artificial ductus arteriosus was created. This increased the amount of blood reaching the lung. As a result, the oxygen saturation of the systemic blood increased and the number of red blood cells decreased.

When the overall methods and results of this research were taken into consideration, it appeared that we had solved the problem of the tetralogy of Fallot or that at least a good beginning had been made toward its solution. As Dr. Taussig had hoped, we, like plumbers, had "changed the pipes" around to get more blood to the lungs. We had found what pipe to put where.[30]

Robert B. Pond, Sr., in a discussion of scientific creativity,[31] stated: "It is completely possible to invent [originate] something and never know what the need is, never know what problem you had solved." It seemed, at this point, that the creation, in 1938, of an artificial ductus arteriosus by Dr. Blalock might well fall into this category. He had then created it and applied it unsuccessfully in attempts to produce pulmonary hypertension in experimental animals.

A tremendous amount of work had gone into this project for over a year. Blood studies had been done on all the animals, red blood cell counts, hemoglobin, and hematocrits. Oxygen content and capacity of arterial blood had been determined. These determinations by the Van Slyke manometric method required approximately 20 minutes each, and all determinations were done in duplicate. If one was able to do the calculations on the previous determinations while doing another, blood gas determinations on each animal would be completed in about 1 ½ hours; otherwise, the time would be nearer 2 hours. There were no oximeters, mass spectrometers, or other electronic devices for the instantaneous determination of the gaseous content of blood in those days. With the normal red blood cell count of about 4,500,000 per square millimeter, counting red cells is time consuming (3 to 5 minutes); in these animals, with counts of 7,000,000 or more, it took even longer. These studies and observations were carried out along with an operative schedule. Clara Belle, a chemistry technician at Hopkins, performed most of the blood studies and assisted in a majority of experimental operative procedures. However, Dr. Blalock had given her the assignment of searching the *Index Medicus* to ascertain if there was anything in the medical literature related to the treatment of the tetralogy of Fallot. She carried out her assignment so religiously and spent so much time in the library that I sometimes found myself operating alone. When I could not manage alone, I would have Tom put on gloves and assist during the more difficult part of a procedure.

The ultimate test of the effect of the anastomosis of the subclavian artery to the pulmonary artery on the tetralogy of Fallot was still to come. There were still unanswered questions. The subclavian artery, the great artery to the forelimb, could be ligated with impunity in a dog. It would sometimes result in a slight temporary weakness of the foreleg, but no long-term or permanent deleterious effects were ever noted. Would a patient tolerate ligation of this vessel? Would the patient with an already diminished flow of blood through the lungs tolerate anesthesia and the occlusion of the right or left pulmonary artery while the anastomosis was being performed? If the operation were tolerated, would the improvement in the general condition of the patient offset any resulting arm weakness? There were no firm answers to these questions.

9

In the latter part of November 1944, Dr. Blalock said that he was going to have to learn to do the subclavian-artery-to-pulmonary-artery anastomosis (creation of an artificial ductus arteriosus) so that he could perform the procedure on a patient. He wanted to assist me in doing one on a dog and then do one or two with my assistance. He came in as scheduled and assisted. He had often observed when I performed various experimental procedures, but he had not participated in them.

On the day he was scheduled to perform the procedure, he telephoned early in the morning. The condition of the patient on whom he planned to operate was deteriorating so rapidly that he could not delay the procedure. He said I should meet with Elizabeth Sherwood, the general operating room supervisor, to go over the instruments he would need and to provide any laboratory equipment that she didn't have.

I promptly went to see Miss Sherwood, who had not yet heard of Dr. Blalock's plans. She had all the necessary instruments for general surgery, even small instruments for pediatric surgery. For vascular surgery, the only thing she had was bulldog clamps (Serrafines) for the temporary occlusion of blood vessels. I actually had little more. She had a great quantity of all kinds of almost any suture material for almost any surgical procedure, except vascular suturing.

Since vascular suture material was not commercially available, the needles had to be threaded with 5-0 braided, treated silk, which was much finer than horse hair. Each operation required four to six sutures. The needles were 1⅛ inches long. In performing an end-to-end anastomosis, the needle length could be tolerated because the vessels could be rotated. The needles, however, were too long to maneuver in performance of the end-to-side procedure of subclavian artery to pulmonary artery. Therefore, they were cut to a length of a little less than ½ inch, on the eye end. Using a spring-type clothespin to hold this eye end of the needle, a new point was honed on each needle with a fine emery block. Cutting, sharpening, and threading needles had been part of my routine for all the experimental vascular procedures that I had been performing, beginning with the coarctation bypass procedure (see fig. 13). I had to inform Dr. Blalock that he would have to use the same type of suture material I had been using.

This had, up to that time, been strictly a laboratory project, and the preparation for the procedure to be done on a patient could hardly be completed in one day. Communication among Dr. Blalock, myself, and the operating-room staff was kept open so that everything was in order; thus the operation was scheduled for November 29, 1944. Suture material had been prepared, and supplies included additional bulldog clamps, a seven-inch straight Adson hemostatic forceps (which was useful as a needle holder), a blunt right-angle nerve hook and smooth bayonet-type forceps to pull up the continuous suture. The clinical teams used the bayonet for this purpose, but I had used it to hold the vessels steady (from the outside) while placing each suture. I did not have good assistants that could be trusted to pull sutures through. These items were all in the general operating room for scouring, packaging, and sterilization.

The morning of the ultimate test of our laboratory efforts arrived. The previous afternoon, Clara Belle had said she intended to observe the procedure in the operating room. I told her I did not think I would go and jokingly added that I might make Dr. Blalock nervous or even worse, he might make me nervous, that he had had me get things ready for him but had said nothing about my being there and that, in any event, from the stands we would not be able to see what was going on. When Dr. Blalock entered the operating room before scrubbing, Clara Belle was already there. He spotted her in the gallery, even though she was capped, gowned, and masked and said, "Miss Puryear, I guess you'd better go call Vivien." On my arrival in the operating room, I went directly to the gallery where Clara Belle was, but immediately the Professor said, "Vivien, you'd better come down here." The patient had been wheeled into the operating room from the adjoining anesthesia room and the skin had been prepped. Dr. William P. Longmire, the Surgical Resident who was to assist in the procedure, was placing the sterile drapes on the patient. The patient was so small, weighing less than 9 pounds, that it was difficult to ascertain whether a patient was beneath the sterile drapes. When all was ready, Dr. Blalock asked me to stand where I could see what he was doing (see fig. 20). The best vantage point was on a step stool placed so that I could look over his right shoulder. Dr. Taussig stood by near the head of the table with the anesthesiologist, Dr. Merel Harmel. The surgical team included Dr. Longmire, Dr. Denton A. Cooley, an intern, and Miss Charlotte Mitchell, the scrub nurse. The chest was entered through an incision in the left fourth interspace. The mediastinal pleura was observed to have numerous collateral vessels giving it a dark bluish red appearance. There was moderate oozing of blood from the mediastinal pleura when it was incised. There were very few specific bleeding points, these numerous vessels being almost capillary in size. Dr. Blalock exposed and then dissected free the left pulmonary artery and passed an umbilical tape beneath it. The pulmonary artery was then temporarily occluded to determine if the patient would tolerate the occlusion. The full length of the left subclavian artery was dissected free. A bulldog clamp was placed at its origin from the aorta, and the vessel ligated as far distal as possible. It was divided proximal to the ligature. The adventitia was stripped from the end of the vessel. The patient's vessels were less than half the size of the vessels of the experimental animals that had been used to develop the procedure. A bulldog clamp was placed proximally on the pulmonary artery. There was a pause to check again the tolerance of the patient to the occlusion of the vessel. A second bulldog clamp was placed

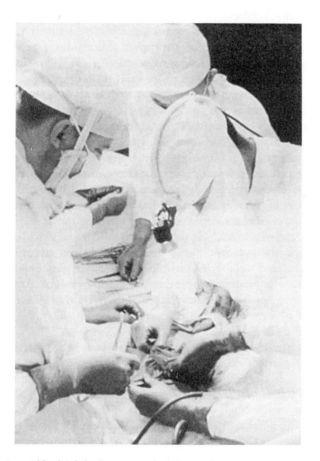

Fig. 20. Dr. Alfred Blalock, at Vanderbilt, performing his first ligation of a patent ductus arteriosus only months after Dr. Robert Gross, of Boston, had first successfully performed the procedure. Courtesy of R. R. Buchholz, M.D.

distally on the pulmonary artery, isolating a segment of the vessel. The patient was tolerating the occlusion. A small transverse incision was made in the isolated segment of the pulmonary artery—the point of no return. Dr. Blalock asked if I thought the transverse incision was long enough; I said I thought it was, if not too long. He began suturing the vessels, starting with the posterior row, which was the most difficult and very tedious. This continuous everting mattress suture was placed loosely. In such small vessels, it was necessary to place each stitch less than one millimeter from the last and very close to the edge of the vessel. When the stitches were in place across the posterior third of the suture line, they were pulled taut by simultaneous traction on both ends of the suture material, thus everting the edges of this segment of the suture line. Stay sutures were placed at each end of the segment and the continuous mattress suture tied to them. A third stay suture was placed in the center of the anterior segment. With slight traction on this, the suturing continued; each stitch was tightened as placed and anchored to the third stay suture, continuing on to the first stay suture, still in place, to which it was tied. With this, the anastomosis of the left subclavian artery to the left pulmonary artery was completed (see fig. 21). The occluding bulldog clamps were removed. There was practically no bleeding. Dr. Blalock was concerned that no thrill was present on palpation of the pulmonary artery. (A thrill results from turbulence when blood from a high or systemic pressure area, such as the subclavian artery, enters a low pressure area, such as the pulmonary artery. It is a sort of buzzing sensation that one can feel with a finger on the vessel. In the closed chest with the use of a stethoscope, it can be heard as a loud noise called a bruit.) He thought the absence of a thrill might have been due to a low systemic blood pressure or to the viscosity of blood from the increased number of red blood cells. The patient was so small that no effort was made to determine the blood pressure. Anxiety in the operating room was somewhat relieved. The chest was closed. Everyone present was pulling for Eileen, the first patient to have the Blue Baby operation, and for Dr. Blalock.

In a letter dated August 5, 1965, to Dr. Mark M. Ravitch, Dr. Longmire, recalling this first Blue Baby operation, wrote: "Vivien Thomas stood in back of Dr. Blalock and offered a number of helpful suggestions in regard to the actual technique of the procedure."[34] The placement of the posterior suture line in this anastomosis is difficult and tedious and, being placed loosely, can be somewhat confusing. In an intestinal anastomosis the sutures are placed to put the outer, smooth peritoneal surfaces in apposition. In a blood-vessel anastomosis, the inner smooth linings or intima of the vessel are placed in apposition by the use of an everting suture. The placing of an inverting or everting suture is determined by the direction in which the needle is passed. Because Dr. Blalock

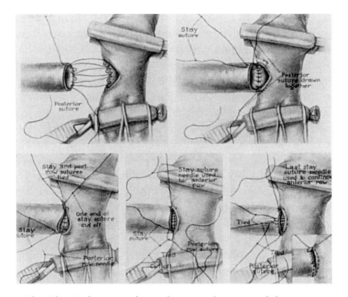

Fig. 21. *The Blue Baby procedure, showing the steps of the anastomosis of the end of the divided subclavian artery to the side of the pulmonary artery. Reading from left to right, top then bottom: a continuous everting suture line is placed loosely on posterior lips. These sutures included entire thickness of both vessels and are approximately 1 mm. apart. The suture is pulled taut, everting the edges of both vessels, and ends of the suture are tied to stay sutures placed at each end of suture line. Anterior suture is pulled taut as placed, interruped at about center and tied to a third stay suture. Last segment of the suture line is tied to first stay suture still in place. The size of the suture material is exaggerated for illustration. Very little of the suture is seen within the lumen of the blood vessels. From Blalock, A.: Surgical procedures employed and anatomical variations encountered in the treatment of congenital pulmonic stenosis,* Surgery, Gynecology & Obstetrics 87:385, October 1948, with permission of Surgery, Gynecology & Obstetrics.

was working on such a small vessel with such fine suture material, I watched closely as each suture was placed. If he began a suture in the wrong direction (which he did on several occasions, having better exposure in one direction than the other), I would say, "the other direction." (On a later patient when I was not watching closely enough, he placed a suture in the wrong direction and, when discovered, whined at me, "Well, you watch and don't let me put them in wrong.") On occasion, he would ask if I thought a particular suture was being placed near enough to the preceding one.

Eileen's recovery was not as smooth or as rapid as we had hoped, but after about two weeks of intensive care, her condition improved. Improvement continued, and after almost two months she was released from the hospital in much better condition than before surgery. Her complexion, no longer ashen blue, was an almost normal pink.

After her discharge, two more patients—a girl, age twelve, and a boy, age six—were operated upon in early February. They were older and in much better physical condition than Eileen had been. Following surgery, there was an appreciable improvement in the condition of the girl and a marked improvement in the condition of the boy.

Everyone involved was excited, happy, and gratified; our efforts in the laboratory were being justified. However, these operations revealed shortcomings that would have to be resolved if this operation were to become a routine clinical procedure. There were no instruments or suitable vascular suture material available commercially. The braided silk that we used was manufactured by J. A. Deknatel and Son, Inc. We contacted the company and inquired as to the possibility of obtaining this fine size braided silk with a swaged-on needle. The vice-president and technical director of the company, Leonard D. Kurtz, M.D., took charge of the inquiry and came to us at Hopkins. He spent quite a bit of time with Dr. Blalock and with me, discussing our needs. Dr. Kurtz, being a physician, may very well have appreciated the significance of this development. For efficiency and ease of maneuvering, a curved needle less than one-half inch long was needed. In a matter of weeks, he had sent us samples of silk with needles swaged on. After receiving approval of silk sizes (4-o, 5-o, and 6-o), needle sizes, and curvatures that would possibly be needed, the company began producing them. Thereafter, there was never a shortage of suture material. They also supplied the laboratory, free of charge, with the suture material with swaged-on needles for our continuing research for several years.

The bulldog clamps used to occlude the vessels were spring-type instruments. The tips had to be tied on beyond the vessels to assure that enough pressure was applied for them to stay in place. The ends of the ties were used for traction in an effort to stabilize the vessels during the anastomosis. After hearing continuous complaints from Dr. Blalock, Dr. Longmire and I decided to have something made that would work better. Louis Miller, a representative of a local surgical supply house, Murray-Baumgartner & Co., met us at the desk in the corridor outside the operating rooms; together, we worked out an instrument using the screw principle on a sliding shaft to exert progressive pressure as the two parallel jaws were brought together to occlude the vessels. This shaft or handle, being rigid, also stabilized the vessels and reduced the transmission of heart pulsations to the suture line. Miller had them made for us in their instrument shop. Dr. Blalock called this instrument the Murray-Baumgartner;[66] today, it is known as the Blalock clamp (fig. 22).

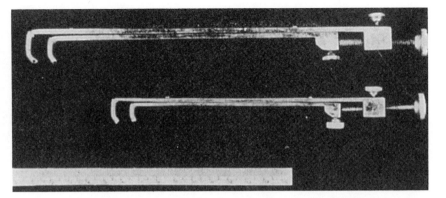

Fig. 22. The Blalock clamp for the temporary occlusion of the pulmonary artery. The long shaft is used to stabilize the vessel. From Blalock, A.: The technique of creation of an artificial ductus arteriosus in the treatment of pulmonic stenosis, Journal of Thoracic Surgery *16:244, June 1947, with permission.*

In the *Journal of the American Medical Association*, May 19, 1945,[28] Drs. Blalock and Taussig described the operation that had been performed on the three patients and gave the postoperative results of the procedure (see fig. 23). A medical reporter read the article fresh off the press; before doctors nationwide had received copies, the story was picked up by the Associated Press and carried throughout the world. Needless to say, Johns Hopkins was not the same for a long time thereafter.

Parents who had Blue Babies read the story. Some went to their doctors, who knew little more than what they had read in the newspapers. Some of the parents did not bother to go to their doctors; they just headed for Hopkins. They came by automobile, train, and plane. Many had not communicated with the hospital, had no appointment in the clinic, and had no hotel reservations; thus the cardiac clinic was overrun with patients. At first they were from all over the United States, but after a few weeks, they began arriving from abroad. To these parents, this operation was their great hope; this was what they had been praying for. I think both Dr. Taussig and Dr. Blalock were greatly surprised by the impact of the announcement. Only three patients had been reported, but the success of the operations and the improvement in the condition of all of them left no doubt in the minds of the parents of these children.

Dr. Taussig had a smooth-running, orderly, efficient procedure for handling patients in the cardiac clinic. There was a moderate patient load, including patients being worked up and studied for possible operation. I had begun, with Dr. Blalock's prompting, to assist her with these patients. About a month postoperatively he had said, "Suppose you get an arterial sample on Eileen. She's on Harriet Lane 4.E." I did not know it,

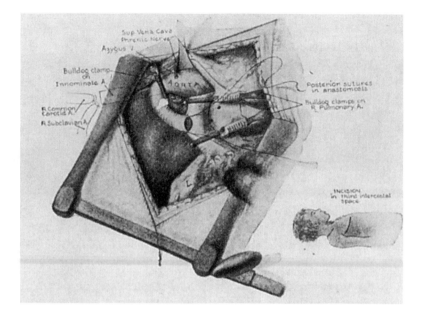

Fig. 23. General exposure of the operative field for the Blue Baby operation on the right side, as presented by Drs. Blalock and Taussig. The end of the innominate artery is being anastomosed to the side of the pulmonary artery. The posterior row of sutures is complete. The anterior row has not yet been inserted. From Blalock, A., and Taussig, H. B.: The surgical treatment of malformations of the heart, Journal of the American Medical Association 128:189, May 1945, copyright 1945, American Medical Association, with permission.

but I had just been elected to do the clinical arterial punctures for the next year. The arterial punctures were performed on the femoral artery as it emerges from beneath the inguinal ligament. At this point, it was easily palpable and fixed so that it had little chance to roll.

When Dr. Taussig had presented the case for Blue Babies in the old Hunterian Laboratory, she had seemed depressed at having to stand helplessly by, watching the condition of these patients deteriorate until they finally died. Her spirits improved when we did the preoperative studies on the second and third patients. Later, when patients began to flood the clinic, she seemed extremely happy. She no longer had to stand by helplessly and acted as if a great burden had been lifted from her shoulders. She never seemed to rush, but she and her staff took care of a tremendous increase in the number of patients seen and diagnosed. Some Blue Babies were not candidates for the operation because they had other abnormalities of the heart in which this procedure would be of no benefit. With an almost uncanny ability, Dr. Taussig was able to differentiate between these patients. Her tools were a stethoscope, an electrocardiogram (EKG), a fluoroscope, and X-rays. The catheterization laboratory was not established until almost a year later.

The operating room was kept so busy that Drs. Blalock and Longmire seemingly stayed there. Dr. Cooley, the intern on the first operation, had rotated to another surgical team. To try to catch up with the sudden backlog of patients, there were two patients scheduled each day, and on at least two occasions, three were scheduled. Dr. Blalock had only done two or three days of this heavy patient load when he was scheduled to be out of town for a few days. Dr. Longmire took over in the operating room and carried on as if this had been a daily, routine operative procedure for months or years. He had had almost as much experience as Dr. Blalock with this particular procedure, having assisted on six or eight cases. Dr. Blalock had observed many but had assisted on only one before he performed his first Blue Baby operation. He had, however, performed some of the end-to-end anastomoses in the kidney and adrenal transplantation projects. He had also sutured a stab wound of the ascending aorta,[14] sutured a stab wound of the left ventricle,[32] and closed the patent ductus arteriosus in patients at Vanderbilt; all performed without the benefit of having had practice sessions in the laboratory, which gave much credence to his native ability as a surgeon. When he returned, I told him how well Dr. Longmire had performed in his absence, and his comment was, "You know he's really good." I agreed 100 percent. Dr. Longmire was one of the very best to go through the surgical residency program at Johns Hopkins during the Blalock era. He had superb natural technical skill, his hands moving deftly, smoothly, and swiftly, and he usually completed the procedure in less time than was required by the Professor.

Not only were patients coming for the operation, but also doctors from all over the United States and from numerous foreign countries came to see the operation being performed by Dr. Blalock and his surgical team. Some of these foreign visitors did not speak or understand English very well. Although usually under constant pressure, Dr. Blalock was always very polite, courteous, and patient with them. I recall one visitor that Dr. Blalock had me talk to because they were having such difficulty getting through to each other. He was very polite during the entire matter, but it was taking too much of his time. I had just as much trouble communicating as Dr. Blalock, but at least I had the time.

The general operating room suite was located on the seventh floor of the dispensary building. The Blue Baby procedure was performed in room 706, which came to be known as the "heart room," or simply 706. In those days, street or civilian clothes were allowed in the operating rooms. Observers or visitors were only required to don a cap and mask and to cover their clothes with a gown. There was a balcony-type observation stand along one side of 706, accessible from the eighth floor above or directly from the floor of the operating room. The operating table was parallel to the stand and less than three feet from it; thus Dr. Blalock and his intern would be almost against the stand. But even from this distance and location, little could be seen. Observers were mostly kept to the stand, but during this period Dr. Blalock would allow one or two of the visiting surgeons on the floor to stand on a step stool for better observation of details of the procedure.

During the first few weeks of the routine performance of the Blue Baby operation, practically every member of the surgical staff came into the operating room to observe the procedure. Even members of the house staff tried to find time to watch. After observing the procedure and leaving the operating room, Dr. William F. Rienhoff, Jr., then an Associate Professor who had been a pioneer in lung surgery, said, "That's not a hard operation, it's easier than an intestinal anastomosis—blood clots." (Obviously he was thinking that a leaking blood-vessel anastomosis might clot and stop leaking, but that a leaking intestinal anastomosis continued leaking and produced peritonitis.)

Lighting was extremely important due to the size of the vessels, the fineness of the suture materials, and the delicacy of the procedure. The large ceiling-mounted light did not give adequate illumination; thus an auxiliary portable spotlight was used. James, the operating room orderly, would focus its concentrated beam, about four inches in diameter, on the exact site of the procedure. This light was on a stand; therefore, the beam could be easily displaced if anyone touched the stand. When this happened, the Professor would literally yell, "Don't move that light." On one occasion, his scrub nurse felt faint and in stepping down from her position, displaced the light. Without looking up, he said, "Don't move that light." The commotion, however, attracted his attention; he looked up and saw the nurse being assisted from the operating room and said, very sympathetically, "Oh, I'm sorry, I wish I could do that some time."

The temperature in the operating room in summer was almost unbearable even to observers. The surgical team, with caps, masks, gowns, and rubber gloves, was often miserable. Often, a circulating nurse stood by, holding a sponge to wipe perspiration from the team's brows so that it wouldn't drip onto the operative field. The great screened windows were wide open—air conditioning in an operating room was unheard of. The Professor used the only available means that would offer a little relief, an electric fan. The fan was adjusted to blow directly on him. If anyone deflected the stream of air, he would immediately order, "Don't get between me and that fan." Everyone in the operating room became extremely conscious of the light and the fan.

Most of the visiting surgeons, often referred to as "visiting firemen" because they usually came in groups of three or four, visited the old Hunterian Laboratory. They came both to see the laboratory where the research had been done and to find out what equipment was necessary to do the experimental procedure in order to go back to their own hospitals, set up a laboratory if necessary, and practice on a few dogs before attempting the operation on patients. There evidently was very little experimental intrathoracic work being done anywhere in the country at the time the Blue Baby operation became a clinical fact. The respirator was a must, so working out an arrangement with Bernard Baker, the chief machinist in Maryland Hall, on the Hopkins Homewood campus, we were able to supply a fair number of them to laboratories around the country.

If Johns Hopkins had a public relations office, it was completely ineffective. Newspaper reporters, especially local ones, were always around. They were in the clinic, in the corridors, and on the patient floors— if they knew where a Blue Baby was located. They would have been in the operating-room suite, except for the ever-watchful eye of Miss Sherwood. To compound this situation, newspapers in different parts of the country campaigned to raise funds to sponsor children from their areas to come to Hopkins. When such a child arrived, there was almost certain to be one of their hometown reporters in the entourage. The influx of patients had developed so rapidly that the Hopkins staff had not set aside or designated any particular area for postoperative care. As a result, patients were in several different areas of the hospital.

Being responsible for doing the arterial punctures for the blood collection and, along with Clara Belle, for the laboratory work on the blood samples, I was put in a particularly awkward position. Dr. Blalock insisted that I look over his shoulder at every procedure he performed in the operating room. If anyone happened to occupy the space where I usually stood, looking over his right shoulder, he would have them move. On one occasion, after some twenty or twenty-five patients had been operated on, I decided to leave the operating room in midoperation. I felt I was wasting my time because questions or comments were seldom directed to me. In one or two instances, after having dissected the subclavian or innominate artery to be used for the anastomosis and pulling down on it with a tape or right-angle clamp, Dr. Blalock asked if I thought it would reach the pulmonary artery to which it was to be anastomosed after it was ligated and divided. Those of us who knew him, of course, felt that in this type of situation he had already decided and knew exactly what he was going to do. On another occasion, because blood samples were needed from several postoperative patients, I had gone to the Harriet Lane Home, which was at least two city blocks away although connected by the long hospital corridor. Before I could collect the first sample, my name came loud and clear over the paging system. I didn't bother to answer the page, but headed for the only place from which it could have originated, room 706. Nothing was said when I entered the operating room. As a result of this incident, I was at Dr. Blalock's shoulder for another twenty-five or thirty cases, when, on my own, I decided not to show up at all. That time he never questioned where I was. I figured that by then surely he knew the answer to any question that might arise. My presence had been mostly for moral support anyway.

Occasionally, there had been an error in diagnosis that would be discovered only after the incision was made, the heart exposed and the size and pulsations of the pulmonary artery observed. The pressure in the pulmonary artery seemed to be high on palpation, possibly Eisenmenger complex. Dr. Blalock wanted to measure the pressure, but there was nothing available that could be used in an aseptic operative field. I proceeded to set up a venous pressure manometer on a meter stick with the necessary stopcock, syringe and connecting tubes. This was wrapped and autoclaved and was in the operating room the following morning. In this type of situation, Dr. Blalock felt more comfortable with me in the operating room. In one of several patients I observed, the measurement of the pulmonary artery pressure was over the 100-centimeter maximum of the water manometer.

Dr. Blalock insisted that arterial oxygen saturation determinations be done on each patient the day before an operation. An occasional arterial sample would be taken in the anesthesia room on Monday on patients scheduled that morning. If we knew ahead of time what patient would be scheduled for the following morning, we would try to complete the determinations and Clara Belle would telephone the results to his office by 5 p.m. Otherwise, I would have the figures in the operating room for him the next morning. I continued to call the operating room at 11 p.m. each night after the schedule for the next morning was posted to be certain he had information on the patient and to be available if needed.

Because no area of the hospital had been designated for the care of these patients, something had to be done. Within a few months Dr. Blalock had a portion of Halsted 3, the children's surgical ward, converted into a ward for the care of pediatric cardiac surgical patients; it was nicknamed the "tet room," because it housed patients with tetralogy of Fallot. A large cubicle in the area was set up as a recovery and intensive care unit. It contained four cribs, the equipment needed to care for the patients and a nurse's desk. At least one nurse was on duty at all times. The other rooms on the floor had two cribs or child-size hospital beds. Many of these rooms would be occupied by the cardiac patients, sometimes as many as twenty or more.

Depending on the group of patients on the floor at a given time, my very presence on the floor would throw the entire floor into an uproar, since it meant that some patient was going to be stuck with a needle. One child would set it off, and in a few minutes every child on the floor would be crying at top voice. If I had the time, I would make extra calls on the floor and talk to the children without getting any blood samples in an effort to change their image of me. There were still a few patients in Harriet Lane across the courtyard and an occasional older patient on other floors.

The hospital did not have a laboratory in which to do the required blood-gas determinations. The arterial oxygen content and saturation had to be done on both preoperative and postoperative patients. Fortunately for us, Clara Belle was still working with us in the laboratory on the clinical determinations. She would spend the first hour each morning preparing the reagents for the blood-gas determinations. These reagents had to be prepared fresh each day, rendered, and stored, air free.

During the first week or so of the deluge of patients, it was a matter of collecting arterial blood samples on patients in the cardiac clinic and performing the oxygen determinations and other studies on them. Then, almost suddenly, things really became hectic because postoperative studies also had to be done. In order not to delay the blood-gas determinations, I usually started about 7 a.m. and collected one or two blood samples from hospitalized postoperative patients before going to the operating room at about 7:30 a.m. Clara Belle and I arranged a pickup point for her to get the samples so that I would not have to return to the laboratory. When the procedure was completed in the operating room, I would go to the cardiac clinic. By this time, several patients would be ready for blood samples to be taken. At first, the clinic patients were all preoperative, but after about three months, there were also patients returning for follow-up studies. From the clinic, I would go back to the wards, where there were other pre- and/or postoperative patients from whom blood samples were to be obtained.

The arterial blood samples for oxygen determinations had to be collected air free. This required especially prepared glass syringes containing an anticoagulant, mineral oil, and lead shot. The lead shot was put in the syringe to mix the anticoagulant with the blood when the syringe was shaken. Hypodermic needles sterilized in glass tubes also had to be prepared. In those days, there were no prepackaged and sterilized disposable needles or syringes. Our material had to be carried along on the rounds for collecting the arterial blood samples. I would not return to the laboratory until at least midday, at which time I would usually relax, drink a Coke, and smoke for ten or fifteen minutes. By this time, Clara Belle would be well along with the oxygen determinations and studies on the early morning blood samples. I would bring in six to eight additional samples so that after having a midday break, it was not unusual for us to be performing the oxygen determinations and the other blood studies until 8 p.m. or later.

Dr. Longmire had been working day and night for about six months on Dr. Blalock's heart team. The past months had been a terrific physical and mental drain on everyone concerned with and involved in the care and treatment of these cardiac patients. A two-and-a-half-year-old girl had never made an attempt to walk or even to stand without coaxing. Her mother broke into tears on entering her room, less than two weeks after the little girl had the Blue Baby operation, to find her standing at the rail of her crib. Scenes like this and seeing the marvelous, almost miraculous improvement in the condition of these little patients with the tetralogy of Fallot, whom we often referred to as "tets," had given all of us the strength and stamina to carry on.

Dr. James M. Mason and Dr. William G. Watson had served successively as chief resident during the first nine months of Dr. Blalock's administration. Broadly speaking, the Professor had inherited these two physicians. As his first free selection of his chief resident in surgery, Dr. Blalock had chosen Dr. Mark M. Ravitch, who held the position from April 1, 1942, through March 31, 1943. On completion of his tenure as chief resident, he went into the armed services and was with the Fifty-sixth General Hospital in the European theater of war. An old friend of mine from Vanderbilt, Dr. Ransom Buchholz, was with the same hospital unit. Returning to Hopkins, Dr. Ravitch again became chief resident. He was trained in cardiovascular surgery by the Professor from December 1, 1945, through January 31, 1946, before joining the full-time surgical staff. He considered Dr. Blalock something of a big brother and, although he accepted a couple of appointments elsewhere, he essentially remained on the surgical staff throughout the Blalock years. In 1969 he settled in as Professor of Surgery at the University of Pittsburgh and Chief of Surgery at Montefiore Hospital.

Dr. Ravitch referred to this present tenure at Hopkins as a "refresher course," but it was actually a new course. He had been away 2½ years and had missed the advent of the exciting new field of cardiovascular surgery and the debut of the Blue Baby operation. Dr. Ravitch's return came at an opportune time to relieve Dr. Longmire as surgical assistant to the Professor. Dr. Longmire had also carried the responsibility of the chief resident since July 4, 1944. In 1948 Dr. Longmire left to become Chief of Surgery and Chairman of the Department of Surgery at the newly established School of Medicine at the University of California at Los Angeles.

10

Late in 1945, Dr. Blalock asked Dr. Richard J. Bing to establish a laboratory to study cardiac physiology. I knew very little of the mechanics of the arrangement, but Dr. Bing and I had fairly close contact. We became good friends while he was setting up the laboratory for the cardiac catheterizations he had planned. The day came when he had his fluoroscopic table on Halsted 3, and the Van Slyke-Neill manometric apparatus for blood-gas determinations (see fig. 24). He had a patient scheduled and asked if I would like to assist him in performing a cardiac catheterization. I told him I would be happy to do so. The nearest I had come to performing cardiac catheterizations was in dogs, in the collection of blood from the right ventricle with the use of a long glass cannula inserted through the external jugular vein in our experimental studies. Plastic tubing had not come into being at that time.

The patient, a four- or five-year-old boy, had been sedated. When we were ready to begin, Dr. Bing suggested that I do the cut-down, saying I, not he, was a surgeon. I accepted his suggestion and proceeded with the cut-down, incised the vein at the inner elbow, passed the catheter a few centimeters into the basilic vein, tightened the ligature around the catheter, and turned the procedure over to him. With both of us watching the fluoroscopic screen, he gently advanced the catheter up the arm until the tip came into view on the screen in the left innominate vein. We then watched as the catheter passed downward through the superior vena cava and into the right aurical. Everything to this point was going as expected. The catheter was supposed to follow the flow of blood from the right auricle to the right ventricle, making a sharp 180-degree turn at the apex of the right ventricle, thence passing into the pulmonary artery. The catheter, as it was advanced, instead of following the expected course, took an abrupt 90-degree left turn from the right auricle and went directly out into the left lung field. We stopped dead still. In the darkened fluoroscopic room, it was difficult to see each other, but I think both of us had broken into a cold sweat. Gently pulling the catheter back into the right auricle, we waited a minute or two and asked the patient if he felt all right.

When the catheter was very gently advanced again, it took the same direction as before. Dr. Bing decided that we should take air-free blood samples for oxygen determination with the tip of the catheter in several

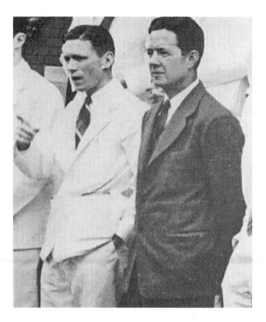

William P. Longmire, Jr., M.D.,
with Dr. Alfred Blalock, 1945

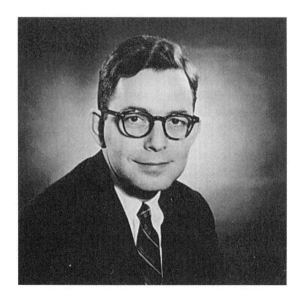

Merel Harmel, M.D.

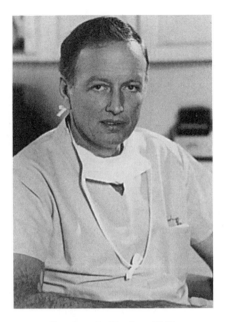

Denton A. Cooley, M.D.

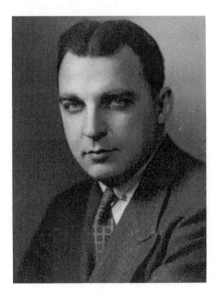

Mark M. Ravitch, M.D.

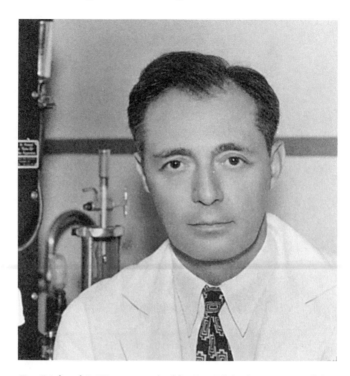

Fig. 24.   Dr. Richard J. Bing was asked by Dr. Blalock to set up a laboratory for the study of cardiac physiology in 1945. He performed the first clinical cardiac catheterizations at Hopkins and developed methods for use of the catheter as a valuable tool in the study of cardiac physiology. He is shown here with the Van Slyke-Neill manometric blood-gas apparatus, which was essential in the determination of the gaseous content of blood.

different locations. The oxygen determinations on these samples indicated that the patient had an interatrial septal defect, through which the catheter had passed. The patient suffered no ill effects from the catheterization. This had been the first cardiac catheterization for Dr. Bing, for me, and for Johns Hopkins.

With a little arm twisting by Dr. Blalock, Dr. Bing and his laboratory personnel took over the patient blood studies that had tied up our research for almost a year. Dr. Bing had been reluctant because he didn't want his laboratory bogged down with these routine studies on cardiac patients. He went on to develop the use of the cardiac catheter as an instrument in the diagnosis and study of cardiac disease and trained many of today's outstanding cardiologists in its use. Dr. Bing is currently

Professor of Medicine at University of Southern California School of Medicine and Director of Experimental Cardiology and Scientific Development at Huntington Institute of Applied Medical Research in Pasadena.

I had observed Dr. Blalock in the general operating rooms on only two occasions prior to the first Blue Baby operation. I was familiar with his demeanor in the laboratory, having worked with him there for years. I was aware of his impatience and tenseness and of how irritable he could be at times, even in the laboratory. Now I had observed him for several months on an almost daily basis in the operating room.

In 706 these traits were magnified to the degree that under stress he seemed to have a different personality. As head of the operating team, he had the greatest responsibility. He was also Chief of Surgery, the Professor, the teacher. He was keenly aware of and extremely sensitive to these responsibilities and did not take them lightly, especially his responsibility to and for the patient. If a patient died on the operating table, it was not unusual for him to leave the hospital for the remainder of the day. If he did not leave, he would sometimes go into his office and become unavailable to anyone.

Dr. Blalock realized and acknowledged the fact that technically he was not the greatest surgeon in the world. Only months after coming to Hopkins, before we had really gotten down to work in the laboratory, he told me that some of the men on the resident staff "could operate circles" around him, but he added that he guessed they should be able to, that some of them were almost as old as he and had spent all day, every day, for the last eight or nine years in the operating rooms. He expressed his feeling that some had been around so long that there wasn't much for them to learn and that space had to be made for younger men who had to be trained.

In the operating room, Dr. Blalock was tense and impatient and, as a result, the atmosphere became tense the moment he entered. Even when things were progressing smoothly he would find something to complain about. Complaining seemed to be a part of him. No one ever seemed to give him sufficient assistance. I was of the opinion that those assisting him were never at their best. Because of Dr. Blalock's tenseness, some were afraid that any move they made might evoke, "Don't do that," or even worse, "Do you know what you are doing?" If the Professor's assistants were not doing exactly as expected, he might say, "This is the same operation, same operation we've been doing every day." He would tell his assistants, "If you can't help me, don't hinder me." His most quoted remark is, "Can't somebody do something to help me?" Such complaints, made in the whining tone of voice that he used when displeased, were enough to have a negative effect on his assistants. Most members of his surgical teams soon learned that these were not particularly derogatory, personally directed remarks. To me, this seemed to be his method of venting some of the pressure he was experiencing. After an outburst, he was often very quiet.

Dr. Blalock was so tense in the operating room that he sometimes got into trouble during an operative procedure. Then he would settle down, relax a little, get out of the difficulty, and quietly complete the procedure without further complication. He seemed to realize that his impatience had caused the problem. Any surgeon can encounter difficulty during an operative procedure; however, the good ones get out of it, and Dr. Blalock was a master at doing so.

To my knowledge, only one operative assistant ever succumbed to Dr. Blalock's outbursts in the operating room. He "froze" and was of practically no assistance to him for the remainder of the operation. After completion of the procedure and partial closure of the incision, I accompanied Dr. Blalock to his dressing room. Lighting a cigarette, he asked, "Did you see that?" I had seen, but asked what he meant. "The way [the assistant] acted," he said. I told him yes, I had noticed. Dr. Blalock commented that he thought everyone knew him well enough not to take him that seriously, that I knew how he was and that the assistant also knew. Saying he guessed he had better apologize, he asked if I thought he should. I agreed that he should, inasmuch as it was so obvious how seriously he had been taken. Dr. Blalock said he would apologize, but doubted that the offended assistant would get very far if he was going to be that sensitive.

Incidents in the "heart room" were widely discussed among members of the surgical house staff; therefore, the surgical assistant should have known what to expect. I had worked with him in the laboratory and thought I knew him pretty well, but his reaction surprised me. He had not been subjected to the worst of the Professor that day. Shortly thereafter, this man with brilliant academic preparation and great surgical ability left academic surgery, but he established a very successful career as a practitioner.

The monthly rotation of surgical teams sometimes caused problems. On the morning of one of the monthly rotations, Dr. Blalock had come into the operating room and had made the incision in the patient's chest. He was about to place the retractor when he suddenly stopped and slowly looked over the team. His first assistant, second assistant, and anesthetist were all new, and his scrub nurse, who usually stayed on the heart team, had a substitute. Still looking around, he calmly asked, "Is there anyone on this team that has ever seen this operation besides me?" Hesitating a moment and getting no response, he stated very matter-of-factly, "Well, that's that. I guess I'll have to do everything myself." Being so absurd, the statement would have sounded humorous to me, except for the pathetic tone of his voice. He settled down to operate, made no complaints, and quietly put on an elegant demonstration of what later came to be known as the Blalock-Taussig operation. As usual, there was nothing lacking in the way of help from his assistants. There was so much cooperation on the Hopkins surgical teams and they were so well trained that if one were to observe only their hands, it might be difficult to differentiate those of the surgeon from those of the assistant.

It became evident team rotation would have to be realigned to accommodate the large cardiac patient load. Dr. Longmire had completed his residency, during which time the Blue Baby era had gotten off to a fast start. Dr. Ravitch had come back for his "refresher course" as chief resident and to be the Professor's assistant, which would only last a few months. Dr. Blalock wanted an assistant resident who would take over and run the heart service without the responsibility of the entire surgical service, which was the chief resident's. Internships were limited to only nine months during the expedited wartime training program. Dr. Cooley had recently completed his internship and Dr. Blalock made him first assistant on the cardiac team while he was still a junior assistant resident. Despite Dr. Cooley's short postdoctoral training, Dr. Blalock could not have made a better choice, considering Cooley's dexterity and technical ability. Until this time, the Professor's first assistant had always been a senior, experienced member of the surgical house staff.

Dr. Cooley was at the other end of the spectrum of personalities from the man who "froze." In one instance, with Dr. Cooley assisting, Dr. Blalock was dissecting to free the right pulmonary artery as it passes posterior to the superior vena cava and the aorta. The patient had not been positioned properly on the operating table and the table had not been rotated; Dr. Blalock was operating from a half-squat position. Dr. Cooley, a six-footer, on a step stool that raised him another six inches from the floor, was nearly standing on his head, his body forming an inverted U in his effort to see the site of the dissection from the opposite side of the table. Dr. Blalock was having a difficult time and was doing a good deal of complaining. Suddenly, he stopped and stood erect. Shaking the instrument in his right hand and stomping his foot, he said to Cooley in a loud, pleading voice, "Come on Denton fella, get on the ball." Dr. Cooley, who by this time was standing erect, towering almost a foot over Dr. Blalock, replied calmly, "Dr. Blalock, I can't even see the ball." The reply broke the tension that had been building. Dr. Blalock relaxed, asked what could be done, had the table rotated, and continued the operation in his normal stance.

Although Dr. Cooley had the utmost respect for Dr. Blalock, he was an independent thinker who had ideas and opinions of his own that he didn't hesitate to express. He always seemed to be comfortable assisting the Professor and did not let Dr. Blalock upset him, even though he, like other assistants, was subjected to verbal outbursts. Evidently Dr. Blalock felt comfortable with him. Now world renowned, Dr. Cooley is presently Surgeon-in-Chief at Texas Heart Institute in Houston.

In the performance of a portal-vein-to-inferior-cava anastomosis, relaxation of the patient is of the essence to obtain and maintain exposure deep in the abdomen. On one such operation, Dr. Blalock had made numerous complaints to his assistants about exposure. He had also complained to the anesthetist about depth of anesthesia and relaxation of the patient. About five or six times he complained to the anesthetist, Dr. Merel Harmel, asking, "Can't you get him a little deeper?" For the fifth or sixth time Harmel replied, "Well, Dr. Blalock, he's pretty deep now." Dr. Blalock stood erect and in desperation said, "Well, if he's that deep, somebody is down in there pushing his guts all over the place." Of course, the patient was more deeply anesthetized immediately. Dr. Harmel is now Professor and Chairman of Anesthesiology at Duke University Medical Center in Durham.

Over the years, the men on the surgical house staff were always fully aware and conscious of the fact that to a large extent their destinies lay in the hands of Dr. Blalock, whose trainees often became professors and chairmen of departments of surgery. They knew he was interested in their present training as well as their futures. At the time of Dr. Blalock's death in 1964, twenty men held such positions or were heads of divisions, mostly the former, in outstanding medical institutions around the country. The Professor took a paternalistic attitude toward them, and the attitude of his overall house staff ran the gamut of son-to-father relationships. These included looking upon him as a good friend or a big brother—with admiration, awe, and utmost respect. If they made it through the surgical residency, they were often referred to as "his boys," which they were, and still are proud to be called. They were intense in their effort to please him, especially if they had any intention of completing their surgical training at Hopkins, which most of them did. The competition was stiff, and they became more and more demanding of those responsible to them as they climbed the ladder to the residency. By the time they completed residency, several were thoroughly disliked by some that had been their subordinates.

In 1945, Dr. Dandy suggested to a medical student, Thomas N. P. Johns, that he talk to Dr. Blalock about the possibility of working in the Hunterian Laboratory that summer. Dr. Blalock assigned him to a project in which he had an acute interest. With vascular surgery having come to the fore, Dr. Arthur H. Blakemore, of New York, a good friend and former classmate of Dr. Blalock, had recently developed and was advocat-

ing the use of an inert metal cannula (Vitallium tube) for use in the anastomosis of blood vessels.[36] Johns, then finishing his third year, was sent to
the laboratory to work with me in an effort to determine if there was any
advantage in the use of these cannulae as compared to the direct suture
technique. Clara Belle and I were performing the blood studies on Blue
Babies, and besides collecting blood samples, I spent part of each morning observing in the operating room. I would take time out during the
afternoon to work with Johns and then rejoin Clara Belle in the patient
blood studies.

In this particular group of experiments, we were to determine how
best to do splenic vein to renal vein anastomoses for the surgical treatment of portal hypertension. We performed end-to-end and end-to-side
anastomoses of the vessels with and without the use of the Blakemore
cannulae. The end-to-side anastomosis tended to remain patent about as
well as the end-to-end anastomoses,[36] and in our hands we found no advantage in the use of the cannulae.

The Blue Baby operation for tetralogy of Fallot was now being performed routinely at Hopkins. However, a procedure for the treatment of
patients with complete transposition of the great vessels had not yet been
developed. Though these patients outwardly presented the same blue or
cyanotic appearance as children with the tetralogy, the circulatory abnormalities were quite different. As had been done in the problem of the
tetralogy, Johns and I began trying to produce the condition (transposition) in order to attempt surgical treatment.

Johns was enthusiastic about the work in the laboratory, where he
took advantage of the opportunity to develop his own surgical skills. He
was the first medical student assigned to work with me on a continuous
daily basis for a period of months. Subsequently, if students participated
sufficiently on any procedure and showed some dexterity and interest,
which most of them did, I would allow them to perform some of the experimental operations while I assisted them. Their demonstration of potential skill and dexterity determined the extent of the operating they
performed. After only a few of the procedures were done, Johns and I began to alternate in being the operator.

Dr. Blalock did not approve of students performing operations in his
research projects. On several occasions when he had entered the laboratory and found me assisting, he told me not to allow anyone else to do the
procedure, that it would throw my results off and that he wanted *my* figures (I called it my batting average). This was not true of Johns, who had
been specifically assigned to the project. It was, however, true with some
of the Fellows (assigned to the laboratory for a year of research), who
came onto the team after the technique for some particular procedure
had been established and a series was in progress. Dr. Blalock would tell

me pointedly that he wanted me to complete the series myself. This was particularly true with some of the more difficult procedures. Most of the Fellows had only finished their internships. They had had much experience as assistants, but had done very little surgery themselves.

Dr. Blalock was anxious to have me in the research laboratory full time, so I returned to the Hunterian after Bing's laboratory took over the routine patient blood studies. There were many cardiac and other problems to be solved, and we had only chipped the tip of the iceberg. A stimulus for further research into the problems of cardiovascular disease, both congenital and acquired, had been provided by the Blue Baby operation, and many problems were being attacked in laboratories across the nation.

There was one question of major concern regarding anastomosing of the subclavian artery to the pulmonary artery in these young patients. What would happen to the size of the anastomoses, the suture lines, as these infants and children grew? Would fibrous tissue in the suture line keep the anastomosis from growing and thus cause a relative constriction of the anastomosis as the subclavian or innominate artery, used for the anastomoses, increased in size?

In an effort to find the answer, a series of anastomoses was performed in puppies, which were smaller than even the first patient. It had always been difficult to raise puppies in a laboratory environment even if nothing was done to them. The average breed of dog reaches full growth in about a year. We tried to use puppies from large breeds in order to have the greatest possible differences of measurements for comparison. Most of the puppies were about 8 weeks old at the time the operations were performed. Six-zero silk was used for the anastomoses. We were working with extremes. The sizes of the subclavian artery in these puppies averaged only two millimeters in diameter.

Operative mortality in the puppies was low, but even with the special care and attention they received, the overall long-term survival was only 22 percent. Autopsy examination of the surviving animals sacrificed at the end of a year revealed an anastomosis with the same diameter as the adult subclavian artery in 30 percent. In 45 percent, the anastomosis was only slightly less in diameter than that of the adult subclavian artery. The suture line in 25 percent showed only a slight increase in the diameter over the measurement in the puppy at the time of operation, each of these having a fibrous ring, a relatively marked constriction. Considering the sizes of the subclavian arteries in these puppies, it was felt that, in dealing with the larger vessels of children, the 25 percent of marked constrictions would be greatly reduced. With today's microsurgery, that 25 percent might have been prevented.

Early in 1946 I was informed by Dr. Blalock of an offer he had received. This time the offer was to become Chairman of the Department of Surgery at Columbia University. Whoever was negotiating with him was making the decision difficult for him. I was not familiar with any administrative problems at Hopkins, nor was I familiar with the finances of the department of surgery. I was, however, familiar with the laboratory and knew we had been operating on a "shoestring," making do with what we had and/or improvising. Dr. Blalock was in an exceptionally good mood the day he informed me of the offer, but did not say that if he accepted, he wanted me to go with him. Instead, he said, "If we go there we will have plenty of money for the laboratory and can do all the research we want to," as if we had an understanding that I was automatically included on any offer he received or accepted. Later, he made a statement to the same effect and seemed so inclined to accept the offer that I told him to include an item in his budget that would enable me to live on Long Island. I had visited New York City just enough to know it was a nice place to visit, and I didn't want to live in Manhattan. Dr. Blalock's final decision, of course, was to remain with his alma mater, Johns Hopkins.

11

Although we had failed in our numerous attempts to produce the cardiac abnormality in the experimental animal, we had, nevertheless, been trying to develop some surgical procedure that might be used to increase the life expectancy of patients with complete transposition of the great vessels—the aorta and the pulmonary artery. In this relatively common congenital malformation of the heart, these vessels have swapped their points of origin. The aorta, which normally carries oxygenated arterial blood to all parts of the body from the left ventricle, arises instead from the right ventricle, which receives unoxygenated venous blood from the body by way of the superior and inferior cavae. The pulmonary artery, which normally carries unoxygenated venous blood from the right ventricle to the lungs to be oxygenated, arises instead from the left ventricle, which receives the oxygenated blood from the lungs by way of the pulmonary veins and left auricle.

This arrangement of vessels essentially sets up two separate circulations: one systemic, in which the right side of the heart recirculates unoxygenated blood throughout the body, the other pulmonary, in which the left side of the heart recirculates oxygenated arterial blood through the lungs. The condition in itself is, of course, incompatible with survival, since no oxygenated blood can get out into the body. These patients, however, do have communications between the two systems, interatrial and/or interventricular septal defects or some combination of anomalies. The size and type of the communications between the two sides of the heart determine the amount of mixing of blood between the systems and thereby the time of survival. The more the mixing, the longer the patient will tolerate the condition and live.

Our thinking at the time suggested getting more oxygenated blood into the right side of the heart, from where it would be pumped directly through the aorta into the general circulation. The right pulmonary veins and right atrium lie in close proximity. Seemingly an easy and simple way to accomplish our aim would be to use a pulmonary vein, which was returning oxygenated blood to the left side of the heart, and reroute it directly into the right atrium.

In these experiments, the right pulmonary vein from the cardiac and apical lobes of the right lung was dissected free along the margins of its attachment to the right auricle. It was then ligated and divided as close as possible to the heart. An opening was made in a segment of the right auricle that had been isolated with a curved clamp. This incision was made long enough to accommodate the pulmonary vein. The free distal end of the vessel was then sutured along the edges of the incision in the auricle, using a continuous everting mattress suture of silk.

When the experimental animals were autopsied, the results were disappointing. The suture line was too often fibrosed, and the vein was constricted. As a result of these findings, subsequent experiments were modified somewhat and greater care was taken in the performance of the procedure. A greater length of vein was obtained, an oval-shaped opening was made in the right auricle, instead of a straight-line incision, and greater care was taken in placing the sutures so as to be certain all edges were everted, thereby placing intima of the vein to the endocardium of the auricle. Much to my dismay, it was found that most of these anastomoses also fibrosed and constricted down from over half an inch in diameter to the size of the lead in a pencil.

The frequency with which these patients with transposition were being seen in the cardiac clinic made this the most urgent problem at the time. Dr. Blalock was taking an intense interest in the project and following it closely. He would often observe these procedures in efforts to determine if there might be some modification of my operative technique that might produce better results.

In order to get sufficient length of the pulmonary vein beyond the confluence of its branches on the right side for the anastomosis to the right auricle, it was necessary to dissect the vein from the atrium. One morning while performing one of these procedures, I noted that I was actually dissecting what I took to be the plane of the interatrial septum. In trying to maintain the thickness of the vein, which at this point contains muscular fibers, I observed a shiny membranous area that I took to be the back surface of the endocardium of the right atrium. If this was truly the interatrial septum I was dealing with, I began wondering if there might not be some way to remove it (see fig. 25). Even a small interatrial defect would allow better mixing of the blood and would surely yield better results than we were presently getting with direct anastomoses.

While proceeding with the operation I had set out to do, my mind was on the removal of the septum. A medical student, Rowena Spencer, scrubbed with me that morning, but I said nothing to her about what was going on in my mind. By the time we completed the operation, I had a good general idea of how to go about the removal of the septum. The big question in my mind was, "What instrument was available for the procedure?" I asked Rowena if she would like to help me "try something" that

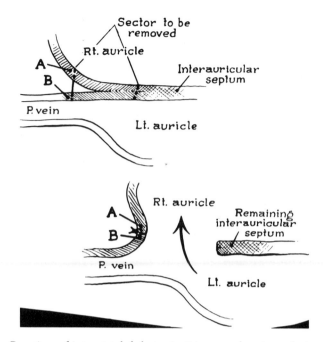

Fig. 25.   Creation of interatrial defects. A: Diagram showing relations between the two atria and the pulmonary vein, which was appreciated in the course of dissecting the pulmonary vein to obtain sufficient length for an anastomosis to the right atrium. B: Diagram of what I thought could be accomplished with the proper instrument, and indeed was accomplished. From Blalock, A., and Hanlon, C. R.: Interatrial septal defect, Surgery, Gynecology & Obstetrics 87:183, August 1948, with permission of Surgery, Gynecology & Obstetrics.

afternoon. She said she had a lecture but would cut it if I wanted her to. There was no full-time research fellow in the laboratory during this period, and I was completely dependent on medical students for assistance.

There was a box of old surgical instruments in the laboratory that dated back to the days of Halsted and Cushing. These were instruments of types I had never seen before, and I had no idea what most of them could have been used for. I rummaged through them during my midday break and came up with an instrument that served the purpose as well as if it had been designed and made to order for what I wanted to try (see fig. 26). I later searched through old instrument catalogs but could not identify it. Rowena returned after lunch and we performed a procedure for the production of an interatrial septal defect under direct vision without interruption of the circulation.

Operations or experimental procedures we think are original with us sometimes turn out to have been done by others years earlier. At that time, this procedure seemed not to have been previously reported or suggested by anyone. In *The Papers of Alfred Blalock*, Dr. Mark M. Ravitch, in 1966, gives it as his understanding that the development of this procedure for the experimental production of an interatrial septal defect had been the result of the observation of a technical misstep by me during an attempt to produce an atrial defect by another technique. With Dr. C. Rollins Hanlon suggesting that "this operative contretemps could be turned to advantage," the account implies that the conception of this method had been that of Hanlon.[34] As I recall and from notes I had written almost immediately following my reading of the Ravitch account, the procedure was developed by my design. My notes dated March 21, 1967, open by stating, "For the sake of the (medical) Archives I am giving my account of the Production of the IASD." The notes further state that after reading the account, "I began to realize how history gets so fouled up." I gave no thought to the possibility that I might make use of the notes myself. With the excitement, enthusiasm, and my own involvement during the early years of the development of cardiovascular surgery, it was an unforgettable experience that is still quite clear in my mind.

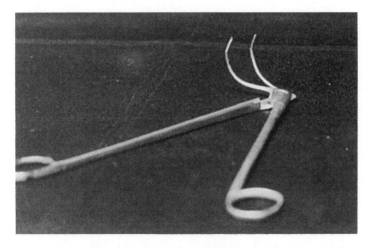

Fig. 26. Unidentified instrument found in the Hunterian Laboratory and used for partial occlusion of the right auricle and right pulmonary vein in the first experimental production of an interatrial septal defect, under vision without interruption of the circulation. The shaft of the instrument is 18 cm. in length, and the effective curved jaws are 3.5 cm. in diameter. There is no ratchet or locking device on the instrument.

For surgery the dog was premedicated hypodermically with ¼ grain morphine sulfate and ⅟₁₅₀ grain atropine sulfate. He was then anesthetized with ether by the open-drop method. After induction, an endotracheal tube with an inflatable cuff was introduced and connected to a positive-pressure anesthesia apparatus.

Aseptic surgical technique was used to make an incision through the right fourth intercostal space. The branches of the right pulmonary vein from the cardiac and apical lobes of the lung were isolated, and each branch was circled with a heavy linen ligature for traction and temporary occlusion. The pericardium was opened along its attachment to the pulmonary veins, extending the incision several centimeters superiorly and inferiorly parallel to the phrenic nerve (see fig. 27). The pericardium was reflected anteriorly and anchored to the chest wall with a suture. The pulmonary artery was then isolated and occluded with a bulldog clamp.

Traction was put on the linen ligatures that had been placed around the branches of the pulmonary veins and each ligature was anchored to the posterior margin of the incision by hemostats. This occluded the veins and gave a good view of the pulmonary vein as it passed behind the right auricle. It was relatively simple with the instrument in hand to pass the lower curved prong behind the vein. The upper prong lay anterior to the

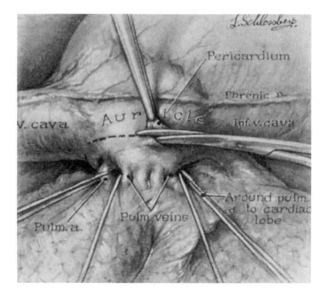

Fig. 27.   Interatrial septal defect. The pericardium is opened along its line of attachment to the pulmonary vein, extending several centimeters superiorly and inferiorly. Traction ligatures around individual pulmonary veins are omitted for clarity. From Blalock, A., and Hanlon, C. R.: Interatrial septal defect, Surgery, Gynecology & Obstetrics *87:183, August 1948, with permission of* Surgery, Gynecology & Obstetrics.

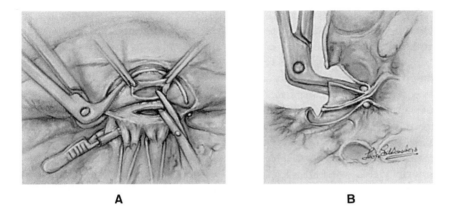

A   **B**

Fig. 28. Interatrial septal defect. The curved occlusion clamp (A) has been placed with its distal jaw behind the left atrium with the proximal jaw in front, thus occluding a segment of both the left and right atria. An incision has been made in the pulmonary vein along its attachment to the right atrium (lower incision). A second incision has been made in the right atrium parallel to the incision in the pulmonary vein. The structure between these two incisions, at tip of scissors, is the interatrial septum. Ligatures around individual branches of pulmonary vein for traction and occlusion and the insrument for traction on the septum are omitted for clarity. Cross-section diagram (B) of clamp in place with segment of interatrial septum isolated for excision. Courtesy of Leon Schlossberg.

right atrium (see fig. 28). The instrument had no ratchet or locking device, so a rubber band was used on the shaft to hold the jaws in approximation. The maneuvers isolated the superior pulmonary vein and a segment of the right atrium. The remainder of the circulation, the superior and inferior vena cavae, the right inferior pulmonary veins, and all circulation of the left side of the heart was left intact and functional.

After applying the partial occlusion instrument, we waited several minutes to see if there would be any untoward effects. There were none, not even a perceptible change in the heart rate. A transverse incision was made in the pulmonary vein for almost its full width on a line about two millimeters from and parallel to the line of its attachment to the right auricle. The only blood to escape when this incision was made was that which had been trapped in the vein by the occluding instrument. Another incision was then made in the right atrium directly opposite and parallel to the one in the vein, about one millimeter from the line of its attachment to the vein. I had been completely convinced, during the dissection that morning, that the structure between those two incisions was a common wall between the right pulmonary vein and the right auricle, therefore, the interatrial septum.

The amount of the septum that could be seen isolated in the clamp between the two incisions was not nearly the amount that I had envisioned being able to remove. But pulling on it with a smooth thumb forceps, I could bring more of it into view. A large curved Kelly hemostat was, therefore, clamped down on it and used for traction. On traction, there was a definite and directional tug on the hemostat with each heart beat and it seemed safe to use this directional tug as a guide for the excision. The first cut, using a curved Metzenbaum scissors, was made superiorly, directly in line of the tug. Then with increased traction on the septum, the inferior and medial cut was made as one continuous cut removing a piece of tissue 1.5 cm. by 1.0 cm. The interatrial septum had been removed, or at least a good portion of it (see fig. 29 B).

The edge of the right atrial incision was then sutured to the remaining edges of the pulmonary vein with a continuous mattress suture of 5-0 braided silk. Care was taken to evert the edges of the vein and atrial wall, in view of the difficulties we were encountering in suturing these structures together (see fig. 29).

The clamp was removed, and traction on the ligatures temporarily occluding the pulmonary veins was released. There was no bleeding, and there had been no loss of blood except that which had been trapped in the isolated segment of pulmonary vein and right atrium. When the bulldog clamp was removed from the pulmonary artery and the heart rate remained constant, I breathed a sigh of relief.

The pericardium was closed with interrupted silk sutures. The lungs were brought to full inflation. The ribs were approximated with heavy linen sutures. (The heavy linen sutures and ligatures used in the laboratory were the same material as that used by shoemakers for stitching on shoe soles, but without the beeswax.) The chest was closed in layers with continuous and interrupted 3-0 silk sutures.

The entire procedure had gone extremely well with none of the complications I had envisioned, and the dog was awake in thirty minutes, although still under the influence of the premedication. Tom Satterfield had given perfect anesthesia. (I had used ether as the anesthetic agent of choice in all the experimental cardiac procedures I had been performing, even though Nembutal was being widely used in the laboratory. Nembutal being an intravenous anesthetic agent, once injected the depth of anesthesia cannot be varied, whereas with ether, administered with a positive-pressure respirator, the depth of anesthesia is easily controlled. Thus, if any difficulty was encountered during a procedure, from hemorrhage or otherwise, and there was a fall in blood pressure, the excess ether could be "blown off" with the oxygen or compressed air.)

Even though the dog looked well enough that afternoon, I was not sure he would survive. Many had been the time that an experimental operative procedure had gone sour overnight. Sometimes an animal may

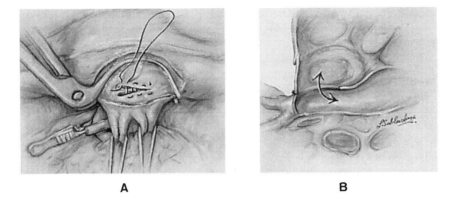

A   **B**

Fig. 29. Interatrial septal defect. With the interatrial septum removed (A), the remaining edge of the incision in the right auricle is sutured to the remaining edge of the incision in the pulmonary vein. One edge of the incision in each had been removed with the interatrial septum. Great care was taken to evert the edges in view of the difficulties we had encountered in suturing these structures together. Cross-section diagram (B) of completed procedure showing interatrial septal defect. Courtesy of Leon Schlossberg.

survive a procedure and you feel encouraged by the immediate outcome, only to come in the following morning and find that rigor mortis has already set in—the operation is a success, but the patient dies. This did not occur in this instance. The dog looked so well the following morning that I decided to do another one. We did another with the same good results, and continued to do still another and another until we had done seven animals with no fatalities. Rowena had assisted on all of them. They were all scheduled and done at a time we knew Dr. Blalock would not walk in. We would check the operating-room schedule, and if he was not scheduled, would wait until after he had made his usual midday visit to the laboratory. The entire procedure only required 1½ hours or less to perform.

The story made the rounds that at about the time for applications for internships, Rowena made an appointment to see the Professor in his office. She had opened the conversation by asking pointedly, "Dr. Blalock, can you give me one good reason I should not have an internship on your surgical service except that I'm a girl?" He must not have had a good one for upon her graduation in 1947, Dr. Rowena Spencer became the first and only female to intern on Dr. Blalock's surgical service. She completed her training as a resident in pediatric surgery in Stockholm, Sweden, and practices pediatric surgery in New Orleans.

I hesitated to let Dr. Blalock know what I was doing, even though I knew he would be deeply interested in this new development. Usually he knew from our conversations and discussions what I was doing and what to expect; I would often make suggestions and inform him of new ideas I might have.

This idea had developed so rapidly and was so appealing that I was eager to determine if it was feasible. If the Professor had made his midday visit to the laboratory that first day, I would most likely have told him about it, even while searching for a suitable instrument. With the very good prospect that it was feasible I immediately scheduled the operation to satisfy my curiosity. One thing I knew for sure was that at whatever point in time he learned of it, he would want to know the results. Therefore, I wanted to wait a sufficient length of time for complete healing to take place before telling him. I felt that he would have been impatient for the results, inasmuch as the transposition problem was of prime interest at the time.

I waited several weeks, then on one of his before-noon visits I told him of the interatrial septal defects we had produced. I showed him my protocols, on which I had shown what I did by making diagrammatic sketches, using a red pencil for those parts of the circulation that carried arterial or oxygenated blood and a blue pencil for the venous or un-oxygenated portion. These sketches had been made on the protocol in which I tried to describe the procedure in the first two experiments. Thereafter, the protocols were only titled "Production of I.A.S.D." (Interatrial Septal Defect) with a reference to the first two protocols. Even now I am not sure I was able to get over to the Professor exactly what had been done.

After about ten minutes of my feeble attempt to explain, Dr. Blalock said, "Let's autopsy one," which, of course, was exactly what I had expected. Having one of the technicians sacrifice the animal on which the first operation had been performed, I went to the autopsy room, removed the heart and lungs intact, and brought the specimen back to the sink in our laboratory. Dr. Blalock was still at the desk in the adjoining office reading the protocols and studying the sketches.

Making no conversation, he came over to the sink, picked up a pair of scissors and forceps and began opening the heart from superior to inferior cavae. At this time, I was all eyes, because I didn't know what he would find, since our mortality had been zero. Neither he nor I spoke for some four or five minutes while he stood there examining the heart, running the tip of his finger back and forth through the moderate-size defect in the atrial septum, feeling the healed edges of the defect. Dr. Blalock finally broke the silence by asking, "Vivien, are you sure you did this?" I answered in the affirmative, and then after a pause he said, "Well, this looks like something the Lord made." We examined the outside of the heart and found the suture line with most of the silk still intact. This was

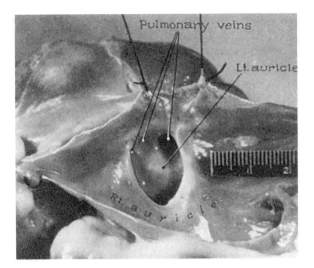

Fig. 30. Interatrial septal defect viewed from right atrium 63 days after operation. Note the left atrium with its entering pulmonary veins, also the smoothly healed edges of the defect. From Blalock, A., and Hanlon, C. R.: Interatrial septal defect, Surgery, Gynecology & Obstetrics 87:183, August 1948, by permission of Surgery, Gynecology & Obstetrics.

the only evidence that an incision had been made in the heart. Internal healing of the incision in the heart was without flaw. The sutures could not be seen from within, and on gross examination the edges of the defect were smooth and covered with endocardium (see fig. 30). We ended the session after performing autopsies on three of the animals on which I had operated. All showed the same good result.

After we had completed the autopsies, Dr. Blalock sat at the desk for thirty minutes or more and wrote up the autopsy notes on the lower part of my protocols.* He began by stating, "This is an operation devised by Vivien . . ." on the first sheet and then went on with his notes.

This method was described by Blalock and Hanlon in a paper in which they gave the results of a series of thirty-one dogs, in which the method was used to produce interatrial septal defects.[37] The preceding account describes the performance and the result of the first operation in that series and how the technique for the production of an interatrial septal defect under direct vision without interruption of the circulation was developed. The procedure was subsequently adopted for clinical use

---

*Unfortunately, these protocols and notes are not available for reproduction as they could have been at the time of publication of *The Papers of Alfred Blalock* by Ravitch, in which reference is made to protocols in my handwriting with a superscript by Dr. Blalock.

in transposition after Dr. Blalock had performed it successfully on animals. He first used it on a patient in May 1948. For a long time it was the only effective palliation for transposition of the great vessels and is still used as the first stage in the Mustard technique for complete correction of transposition, although largely supplanted by the angiographically controlled cardiac catheter balloon septostomy.

When his notes were completed, Dr. Blalock asked me to do the procedure while he assisted so that he could see exactly how it was done. Next morning I did so; and everything went smoothly. However, he didn't like the instrument we were using, especially because a rubber band had been used to approximate the jaws, and asked if a better one could be made. William O. Jones, an expert machinist employed by the Medical School, was consulted; together, we devised an instrument with a spring in the handle, which exerted constant pressure on the movable upper jaw against the lower fixed jaw (see fig. 31). This instrument was used on the first clinical case, but was then redesigned so that the amount of pressure exerted by the jaws could be adjusted. Dr. Blalock also thought that I should run the series of experiments up to about twenty animals, which I did in the next several weeks.

I worked with Leon Schlossberg, who illustrated the procedure for publication. With innate talent and ability, Schlossberg, a student of the

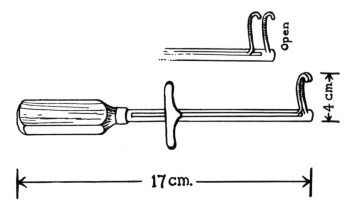

Fig. 31.   *Instrument for use in the production of an interatrial septal defect. Dr. Blalock had assisted in the demonstration of the production of an interatrial septal defect using the unidentified instrument shown in fig. 26. The above instrument has a compression spring in the handle that exerts pressure on the upper movable jaw against the lower fixed jaw. The pressure exerted by the spring could not be adjusted and the instrument was redesigned. From Hanlon, C. R., and Blalock, A.: Complete transposition of the aorta and pulmonary artery, Annals of Surgery 127:385, March 1948, with permission.*

late Max Broedel, was, at least to us at Hopkins, the most outstanding medical illustrator in the field. An academic degree in art, which is now required, was not mandatory; thus Schlossberg, in 1931, began his three-year study of art as applied to medicine. Upon completion, he remained at Hopkins as a free-lance medical illustrator. On his arrival at Hopkins in 1941, Dr. Blalock showed interest in Schlossberg. In 1942 Schlossberg was called into the armed services and served as Officer in charge of Medical Illustration at the Naval Medical Center, Bethesda, Maryland. Upon his discharge in 1946, he returned to Hopkins, where Dr. Blalock and others on the surgical staff began using his talent. To be certain that Schlossberg was available to him and others on the surgical staff at all times, Dr. Blalock, in 1952, assigned him a room on the sixth floor of the newly erected building, now known as the Blalock Clinical Science Building. Here the entire full-time surgical staff was located, and here Schlossberg produced the fabulous and superbly vivid illustrations in the Blalock publications and in the publications of many others in the department of surgery. His talent continues to be sought by former Hopkins surgeons now at other institutions, such as Henry Bahnson, A. Glenn Morrow, and Mark Ravitch. Aside from his medical illustrations, he has made models of the heart[38] and of the human skeleton,[39] both for teaching and commercial use. He has also published the *Atlas of Human Functional Anatomy*, with text by George D. Zuidema, M.D.[40] Schlossberg is Assistant Professor in the department of art as applied to medicine, at Hopkins. He recently recalled his difficulty in illustrating the interatrial septal defects to Dr. Blalock's satisfaction.

In developing his illustrations, relationships between structures had to be defined. For this, the heart and lungs were isolated by tying off the aorta and the superior and inferior cavae. All blood was removed from this isolated portion of the circulation. The heart and lungs were then filled with an injection of 10 percent formalin at a pressure of about 75 mm./Hg., and the lungs were inflated to their normal position. The preparation was left overnight to fix. The heart, with its great vessels intact, was removed. With a large butcher knife, it was then sectioned from base to apex, thus giving a good sectional view of the entire heart, the ventricular and auricular walls, and the septae dividing the right and left chambers.

This was essentially the method I'd used to learn anatomy during my early years in the laboratory at Vanderbilt. After many months of studies on shock, we began performing experimental surgical procedures. I knew it would be to my advantage and thought that it would be interesting to learn the anatomy of the dog in this manner. Blood for transfusions in ongoing studies on shock was obtained by bleeding out the donor. Organs and other structures always shift or move from their normal position if dissections are carried out in live or freshly dead animals. On numerous occasions, I would embalm the donor with fluid obtained from William "Bill" Gunter in the autopsy room; thus all organs would be fixed *in situ*. The animal would then be wrapped in a moistened gown and kept in the walk-in refrigerator. As time permitted, I would dissect these embalmed specimens, determining exact anatomical position of organs, their blood supply, and their relative position to each other. I would also dissect and section the individual organs.

In the fall of 1946, Rowena Spencer returned to the laboratory to assist whenever time permitted. Dr. Blalock had me schedule the procedure for producing an interatrial septal defect so that Dr. C. Rollins Hanlon could observe. I had not met him before, but he was to work closely with us until 1950, when he would leave Hopkins to become Professor of Surgery at Saint Louis University. After checking to see if we were ready in the operating room, Dr. Blalock took Hanlon to our laboratory and showed him specimens from the animals with atrial defects on which he had already performed autopsies. Hanlon evidently understood the technique of the procedure because during the demonstration, while looking over my shoulder, he suggested I excise the septum more superiorly in order to remove a larger segment of it. I did so while he instructed. (Following the demonstration of the procedure on which he assisted the day after the three original autopsies, Dr. Blalock had asked if it was possible to make the defect larger and if so I should try.) The remaining part of the procedure was carried out in the same manner as the previous ones. Removal of the curved occlusion clamp resulted in profuse bleeding that was impossible to control with sutures. The origin of the bleeding was located too far posteriorly. Autopsy revealed that the superior excision had extended beyond the line of fusion of the pulmonary vein and the right auricular wall. The hole or opening was thus in the outer wall of the auricle. This had been my first fatality.

Hanlon and I became closely associated in research and in the administration of the laboratory. He took an active role in the cardiac research, but only occasionally did we work together as a surgical team. He modified the technique of the original shunting procedure and completed the series of experiments I had been doing—that is, the shunting of the pulmonary vein blood directly into the right auricle (see fig. 32). He instead shunted the blood from the pulmonary vein through an enlarged orifice of the azygos vein into the superior vena cava, which gave a smoother surface for the suturing than did the right auricle (see fig. 33). His results (pulmonary vein to superior vena cava) were almost 80 percent patencies (see fig. 34), whereas ours (pulmonary vein to right auricle) had been

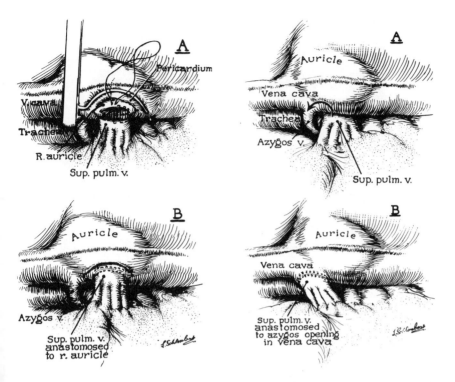

Fig. 32. *In experiments on the treatment of transposition of the great vessels, the right pulmonary vein is anastomosed to the right atrium. A: Clamp prevents bleeding from right atrium while anastomosis of right pulmonary vein is being made to an oval opening in the atrium. During dissection to obtain sufficient length of the vein, I noted that the anterior wall of the vein fused with the posterior wall of the atrium to form the atrial septum (fig. 25) and conceive a method for production of the interatrial septal defect. The clamp shown in the illustration had not been devised when this series of procedures was first begun. Bulldog clamps to prevent backflow of blood from the lung are omitted for clarity. B: Completed anastomosis of pulmonary vein to right auricle. From Hanlon, C. R., and Blalock, A.: Complete transposition of the aorta and pulmonary artery, Annals of Surgery 127:385, March 1948, with permission.*

Fig. 33. *Hanlon modification of treatment of transposition of the great vessels. Anastomosis of the pulmonary vein to the superior vena cava. A: Vessels in normal position with arrow indicating proposed site of anastomosis to an enlarged orifice of the azygos vein. B: Completed anastomosis. From Hanlon, C. R., and Blalock, A.: Complete transposition of the aorta and pulmonary artery, Annals of Surgery 127:385, March 1948, with permission.*

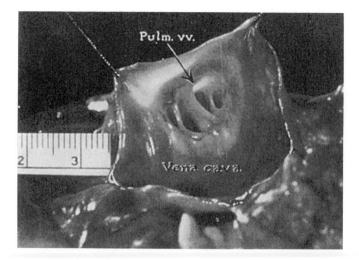

Fig. 34. *Anastomosis of superior pulmonary vein to superior vena cava. Superior vena cava opened to show smooth healing 83 days after anastomosis of superior pulmonary vein to vena cava. The anastomoses were 80 percent successful. From Hanlon, C. R., and Blalock, A.: Complete transposition of the aorta and pulmonary artery,* Annals of Surgery *127:385, March 1948, with permission.*

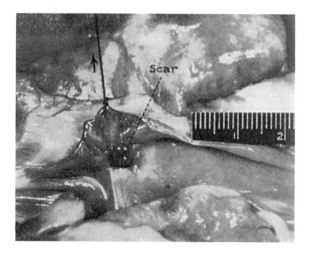

Fig. 35. *Right auricle opened to show hyperplastic scar at the site of an unsuccessful anastomosis of the superior pulmonary vein to the right auricle. Such anastomoses were only 20 percent successful. From Hanlon, C. R., and Blalock, A.: Complete transposition of the aorta and pulmonary artery,* Annals of Surgery *127:385, March 1948, with permission.*

slightly less than 20 percent satisfactory (see fig. 35). Detailed descriptions and results of these shunts were reported by Blalock and Hanlon.[41]

Years later, on the occasion of the presentation of my portrait, it was Dr. Hanlon who made the warm and laudatory presentation speech. In my remarks, I spoke of what great friends we were and of how kind he had been to include me as co-author of one of his papers.[29] However, I could not resist the temptation to add that I thought he should have included me in two. I had expected some reaction to the comment, but was surprised by the amount of laughter and applause from those in the audience who knew I was referring to the operation for transposition.[37]

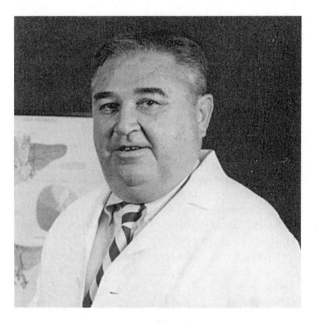

Leon Schlossberg

12

After World War II ended, in 1946, we had a chance to take our first vacation since arriving in Baltimore in 1941. My wife and I, with our children, headed for Nashville. We were not natives of Baltimore, thus we were happy to head home to see family and old friends. If things looked promising economically in Nashville, consideration might be given to returning. The war had brought most civilian production to a grinding halt. Everything was in short supply, including housing. Now the war was over and the postwar boom was on, including the building trade.

Both my father and a brother, who were still in the trade, had more jobs than they could handle. I talked with them and many others I knew in the trade, and seemingly everyone was in the same situation. My father offered to let me fill the contract on a house he had not even started. Almost everyone I talked with was ready to give me a job then and there. There simply were not enough carpenters to meet the demand. It was quite a temptation but required much more thought and consideration.

I talked with our tenant, an employee of Vanderbilt, and told him his lease probably would not be renewed the following year. Knowing Dr. Blalock and our relationship in the laboratory, he laughed and said, "I'm not worried. Dr. Blalock isn't going to let you come back here even if he has to pay you out of his own pocket."

Leaving Nashville, we then went to Macon, Georgia, my wife's former home, to visit her family and friends and to relax. The visit to Nashville had turned out to be a work and business trip.

Upon returning to Baltimore after vacation, I had many conversations with my wife about what to do. The decision was finally made the latter part of October, and only the details of the move had to be worked out. Wanting Dr. Blalock to know of our plans, in early November I told him we were planning to move back to Nashville the following spring. I let him know then because I thought he would want me to train a replacement or, more likely, find a full-time physician who knew some surgery and would be interested in research to carry on his work. I told him I planned to leave around April and that Clara would stay in Baltimore until the children finished the school year.

Our dialog went essentially like this:

BLALOCK: What's the matter, don't you like it here?

THOMAS: I don't have anything against the place, but I still have the children to look out for. In about five years the older one will be coming out of high school and be ready to go to college. I want to give them a better chance than I had and give them as much education as they want, but I won't be able to if I stay here at Hopkins.

BLALOCK: (whining) Well, Vivien, you're making more money now than anyone around here without a degree. (The Professor, not usually on the defensive, had been surprised by my announcement.)

THOMAS: That's the problem, that's the reason I plan to be able to let my children get all the degrees they want. Hopkins has a pay scale and I fall within a certain salary bracket. I don't have a degree so that I can get a promotion and be up-graded for better pay. I'm not even asking for more money here. I've just gone ahead and made my plans to get it elsewhere.

BLALOCK: What do you plan to do?

THOMAS: The only other thing I know anything about. Go back into the building trade.

BLALOCK: (smiling) I'll bet you can't even drive a nail straight by now. How much do you figure you can make?

THOMAS: Oh, anywhere from two to four times what I'm making here. Maybe more, depending on how hard I want to work or how much I hustle.

BLALOCK: Well, you aren't leaving tomorrow, so we'll have plenty of time to talk.

The Hopkins Medical School did not pay for overtime. Employees were theoretically supposed to receive compensatory time off. I say theoretically because no one but those associated with Dr. Blalock would appreciate the difficulties that would be encountered in attempting to get compensatory time from him. The official work week was 37½ hours. On coming to Hopkins, he had complained that "people here don't start to work until nine o'clock," by which time he considered half of the day gone. Medical School hours were from 9 a.m. to 5 p.m. with an hour for lunch and from 9 a.m. to 11:30 a.m. on Saturdays. At Vanderbilt, the hours were from 8 a.m. to 5 p.m. daily and from 8 a.m. to 12 noon on Saturdays, a 44-hour work week. At Hopkins, the University and the Hospital are separate institutions, each having its own board of trustees and administrative staffs. The hours for the School of Medicine are set by the University, of which it is a part. The schedule of hours applied to the administrative staff, secretaries (the Professor's secretaries were University employees), the technicians, and all personnel on the Medical School grounds. Dr. Blalock was coming in at 7:30 to 7:45 each morning, and if he wasn't operating, which began at 8 a.m., he was essentially lost until 9 o'clock when the secretaries came in. With the ten- to fourteen-hour shock studies and the twelve- to fourteen-hour days during my clinical involvement in the Blue Baby operation—and, on occasion, taking paper work home with me—I had averaged nearly sixty hours a week over the past five years. I was never asked directly to work the longer hours and made no attempt to negotiate for compensatory time. The Professor had a way of getting the most from everyone around him, without their realizing how hard or how long they were working. I was aware and didn't mind, but economically, with no overtime being paid, something had to be done. Dr. Blalock had asked how much money I expected to make elsewhere. To work those hours I surely would make no less than I was making at Hopkins. To Dr. Blalock, one lived to work and the work day was twenty-four hours long with a little time out to sleep. For the surgical house staff, there was very little time for that (see fig. 36). I was satisfied and deeply interested in my work. In fact, I thoroughly enjoyed it, but I had the responsibility of my family and felt it my duty to see to their future welfare and mine.

Several days later, Dr. Blalock and I had a long discussion in which he made alternative suggestions. However, he made no salary offer. Laboratory work continued and he made his usual visits. About two weeks later he made a salary offer. I told him either he was kidding or he thought I was—the amount of his offer would barely let us break even. We already had a little extra income from the rent of our house in Nashville. This was his first knowledge of the house and some discussion about it followed. I told him that Robert (Bob) Sanders, a former patient of his, lived in the house and that I had served notice on him. He remembered him and asked how he had been getting along. Dr. Blalock had been instrumental in getting Bob Sanders the job at Vanderbilt after having performed a thoracoplasty on him. I told him we probably would have already left if my wife had not been such an efficient manager, homemaker, and seamstress.

Two more weeks passed before he made another salary offer, which was much better but not good enough. When I turned it down he made such a fuss and asked what I expected that I had to remind him I wasn't asking for anything, he was making offers I hadn't asked for, and I didn't want Hopkins to break their rules. I was thirty-six years old and if I had

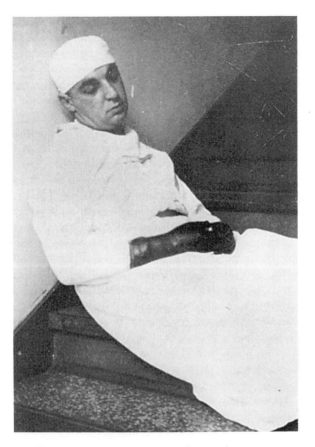

Fig. 36. Mark M. Ravitch asleep on steps of general operating room. With the staff and house staff depleted by war-time departures, and the duties and responsibilities of the resident increased under the Blalock regime, time between cases had to be profitably employed. Courtesy of Robert S. Sparkman, M.D.

to change jobs, I should do so before I was forty. Furthermore, I didn't see Hopkins or the medical field as the place for me without having a medical degree if we were to live comfortably and educate our children. I also told him about friends and acquaintances who were doing very well without degrees, thus I could do the same.

After our conversation that day, I didn't think he'd ever mention it again. I did most of the talking, but we were both emotional and tense. He was disappointed that I didn't accept his offer, but my decision to make the change was so firm that I would have preferred that he not make an offer. I felt he was interfering with my personal plans and affairs.

The research continued for three weeks as if nothing was going on behind the scenes. We were approaching Christmas, so I had decided the whole thing was over. However, I had grossly underestimated the extent to which Dr. Blalock would go to get what or whom he wanted. Only those who knew him or had occasion to hear his tone of voice under certain circumstances can appreciate when I say he'd whined during most of these sessions.

Two or three days before Christmas, I received a call from Dr. Blalock just before noon. He said he was glad he'd caught me. Knowing everyone would be leaving for the holidays at noon, he asked if everyone had gone. He wanted to see me and asked that I stay around, that he would come over in about half an hour. I hadn't seen him in several days and thought he might want a thorough update of the research work prior to the holidays, during which time he liked to think and study.

When he arrived and was assured that everyone had gone, he said, "Good, we've got to have a talk." We went into the office and sat down, which was unusual, so I thought, "Here we go again." He hesitated, then began in a calm, slow, easy tone of voice. "Vivien, I've done something on my own and I hope it will interest you. I've been working with Dr. Chesney [Dean of the School of Medicine], trying to work out something about your salary. He has been very sympathetic and cooperative. I've made a recommendation, which he carried out to Homewood this morning. The Board of Regents [trustees] has approved it and Dr. Chesney has just brought it back." He reached into his pocket and pulled out a file card on which some figures were written. Passing it to me he said, "I hope you will accept this—it's the best I can do, it's all I can do."

There were two dates on the card, January 1 and July 1, with dollar figures beside each. When I read the figures on the card, I was flabbergasted. The figure beside January 1 was more than his most recent annual salary offer. For July 1, it was almost twice my salary at the time. Was Hopkins really making me this kind of offer? I sat so long just looking at the card, he finally asked, "Well, what do you think?" Getting up from where I was sitting, I told him it was hard to think, that this was quite a shock. I asked when he wanted an answer and he said he would like it that day, immediately if I could decide. I went down the hallway, got a Coke from the machine and went to the phone at the far end of the building.

I called my wife and told her what was going on, but she left the decision entirely to me. I had to perform a lot of mental acrobatics figuring the pros and cons of the situation. Dr. Blalock was entertaining himself with the protocols and notes of his experiments on the desk in the office. After about half an hour of pacing the floor, I returned to the office and told him I would accept the offer. He then told me there was one condition: the subject of my salary could never be brought up again. If I made any further demands, I would have to leave. I tensed at the use of the word *demand*, but took a deep breath and didn't say anything for a moment; then I stated very calmly, "I think you should have given me the condition in the first place. One thing I would like to get straight is that I have not made any demands on anyone, not on you or the University." He interrupted, "Well, if you become dissatisfied with your salary," but I broke in, "This puts a whole new thinking in the picture. I already have my plans that can still be carried out. I can't afford to get stuck, even at the salary you are offering unless it's in a new salary bracket they have established and these figures are near the lower end of that bracket."

I finally told him that I would accept the offer and he could depend on me for the next year and a half, which was covered in the offer. After that, if I ever found myself in a financial bind, I would give him a thirty-day notice with no negotiations from either side, because I didn't want to go through anything like this again. There was silence for a few moments, then he asked, "But you will stay now?" I said yes. Then, with the smile of a victor, he said, "Thank God, that's over. Maybe we can get some work done now." I told him I had been working the whole time.

In leaving, he wished me and my family merry Christmas; walking briskly down the hall, he called back, "Don't forget to tell Bob he won't have to move." I thought about Bob's remark that Dr. Blalock would pay me out of his own pocket and wondered what would have happened if the trustees had turned down his recommendation. As it turned out, I was placed in the lower end of a newly established salary bracket for non-degreed personnel who deserved a higher pay scale.

As a result of this episode, our older daughter, Olga T. Norris, received her bachelor's degree from Morgan State College, now Morgan State University, in 1956. She spent a year with Dr. Curt P. Richter in his laboratory. Later, she went to the department of otolaryngology as a histology technician with Robert J. Ruben, M.D.; Diran O. Mikaelian, M.D.; and Dickens Warfield, Ph.D. In 1965, both Ruben and Makaelian left the institution, but Olga and Warfield felt that the project on which they were working was sufficiently important to complete. As volunteers, they completed the project in the otophysiology laboratory over the following six months, and the study was eventually published.[42] Olga now has a lucrative hobby in arts and crafts. Ruben is Professor and Chairman of Otolaryngology at Montefiore Medical Center and Albert Einstein Medical School.

Our younger daughter, Theodosia T. Rasberry, opted for business education at Cortez-Peters Business School. Having taken additional studies at Morgan State and at the College of Notre Dame of Maryland, she is Publication Specialist with the U.S. Department of Health and Human Services.

After I had first informed Dr. Blalock of my plans to leave Hopkins, he tried to influence my thinking about leaving. He didn't think the building boom would last more than three or four years and asked what I would do if this happened. I told him I would do all right and it was a chance I'd have to take. I said I didn't know what would happen if I left Hopkins, but I knew what would happen if I stayed. He asked if I thought I might be willing to come back to the laboratory if things went badly in Nashville. I told him I didn't know and would make no commitment. He was aware, of course, that for additional income I was moonlighting as bartender for house parties given by the professional staff, his parties included. He was concerned that if I ever left town I wouldn't return and asked why I couldn't find another job in Baltimore rather than leave town. To this, I replied that rent was a big item from one's income, and in my plans I would not have to pay rent. He finally suggested that, in addition to whatever salary increase he might offer, I should be able to subsidize my salary while still working in the laboratory. He explained that I was buying a large dollar volume of laboratory supplies, that there was considerable mark-up from the vendors, and that salesmen get a good commission. He didn't see why I couldn't make direct contact with some of our suppliers, cut out the salesmen, and collect the commissions myself. He thought I might even make contacts with other laboratories around the Medical School. He had seen several salesmen in my office on his visits to the laboratory and, knowing my negotiating tactics, thought I could even save money for the laboratory by dealing direct. He didn't see anything wrong in doing such a thing, as long as the prices were kept competitive. If I did make such an arrangement, he didn't want to know about it; then he smiled and said I'd probably make so much money that he might want a cut of the commissions. Even though I would have been a bona fide salesman, such an arrangement, by today's code of ethics, would, of couse, be classified as a conflict of interest.

I immediately gave serious consideration to Dr. Blalock's suggestion, since I would've needed the extra money to move back to Nashville. I had defrayed my own expenses to move to Baltimore. Salesmen make friends if they are to stay in business, and several major suppliers and I had become fairly good friends. They were men like myself with families, trying to make an honest living. It seemed almost unconscionable to me to undercut these men.

I had had a medical problem during our first year in Baltimore and, not knowing any physicians in town, had talked to Dr. Blalock about it. He told me that if I wanted my own private physician, I should see Dr. Ralph J. Young, "the best doctor in town, colored or white" (see fig. 37).

I went to see him and we almost immediately formed a close and lasting friendship. In his mid fifties, Dr. Young had slightly gray, thinning hair; he was chubby, but not fat, with a pleasant personality. He was jovial by nature, but very serious when the occasion warranted it. He was one of the last of the "family doctors" and one of the last to stop making house calls, which he did because of age and health. His office hours, except for

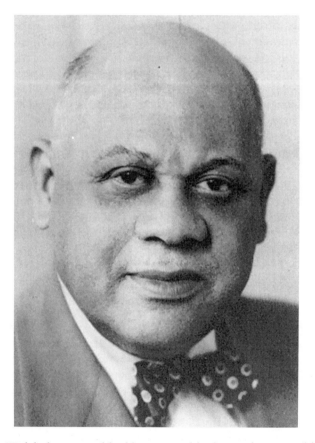

Fig. 37. Widely known and highly respected by his profession and by laymen, Dr. Ralph J. Young was dedicated to the care of his patients. He was recommended to me by Dr. Blalock in 1942 as being the best doctor in town, colored or white. Johns Hopkins eventually appointed him to the hospital staff in 1946 and to the university faculty in 1952. Courtesy of Moorland-Springarn Research Center, Howard University.

house calls, were almost continuous, and he seldom left his office until 11 or 12 o'clock at night. His wife often sent meals to his office. His life was dedicated to the care of his patients, to the extent that he continued to see them against his own doctor's advice, even after he had suffered two myocardial infarctions.

On a visit at his home during recuperation from his second heart attack, I asked why he didn't retire and stop driving himself. He replied in his usual jovial manner, "You think I'm just going to sit here and wait for 'The Man' to tap me on the shoulders? No, I'm going to see my patients as long as I can get around." He was highly respected in his profession for his diagnostic acuity; most of his patients, with utmost confidence, felt they could live forever if he was around to care for them. He died November 15, 1968, at the age of seventy-five. He had lived up to Dr. Blalock's assessment of him. To my family and me, Dr. Young had been friend, father, counselor, advisor, and doctor. His only child, a daughter, Lois A. Young, graduated from the University of Maryland Medical School in 1960, was on the opthalmology staff at Hopkins for one year, 1965–66, and is currently at the University of Maryland Hospital as Associate Professor of Ophthalmology.

Because Dr. Young had known of my plans to leave Hopkins before Dr. Blalock, I had consulted with him about Dr. Blalock's suggestion. Dr. Young's sympathies were divided. He understood the situation my family and I were in, but he was connected with the Hopkins medical institutions, being the only Negro physician working in their clinic; thus I could understand and appreciate his feelings. He and I were both firsts in our respective positions at Hopkins. In 1946 Dr. Young received an appointment to the regular hospital staff; in 1952 he was appointed to the Medical School faculty.

Dr. Young was paying careful attention as I related to him the conversation I'd had with Dr. Blalock. I told him of my feelings toward the displacement of salesmen with whom I dealt. He went down his mental list of companies and salesmen and finally mentioned the name of a company with which I had not dealt; A. J. Buck and Son was essentially a veterinary supply house, but also handled a large line of doctors' office supplies and equipment. As instructed, I went to see the manager, whose name I can't recall. I introduced myself by name only and told him that he had been recommended to me by Dr. Young. I told him that I had some contacts and that I thought I might be able to make some contribution to his company, if I were allowed to act as a salesman. He asked how much money I wanted. I told him I didn't want anything but a salesman's commission, only on what I sold. He told me there was no way I could help his company, that he had just about every colored doctor in town on his customer list, that they were all his friends and that he already had one of his men calling on them. I told him I didn't have doctors' offices in mind. He didn't inquire, so I didn't feel it advisable to name my contacts since in his judgment a salesman or a representative of his company was known by his skin color rather than by the dollars he might bring into his organization. In leaving, I asked again if he was sure he didn't want an increase in his sales. Smiling and courteous, he replied, "No, you can't do anything to help us." This attitude was a sad state of affairs, but unfortunately it was common at the time.

About three years later, a salesman for A. J. Buck and Son came into my office and introduced himself. I offered him a seat by the desk and listened attentively as he listed the items he thought he could supply our laboratory, and I even asked a few questions. Then I related to him the conversation that had taken place in the office of his company three years earlier, telling him that his company could have had the lion's share of our business then, that it would have amounted to possibly tens of thousands of dollars since that time, but as far as I was concerned it would stay where it had been put on that occasion. I had made the offer and it had been refused; thus the offer had been withdrawn. I told him there was no feeling in the matter as far as he, as an individual, was concerned, but for him to be sure to tell the folks in the office, especially his boss, to be careful of what they say to people who come in off the street, that it can make it mighty tough on the salesman who has to go out there.

After my failed attempt to become a salesman, Dr. Young referred me to Dr. Ben Gaboff, a pharmacist, who was president of a relatively small local concern manufacturing a few pharmaceuticals, the Ralph Winton Company. Dr. Young talked to Gaboff before I contacted him. Gaboff was interested in a Negro as a "detail man" to contact the Negro doctors in Baltimore and introduce company products. The purpose in this effort was to have the doctors prescribe the products to their patients.

I went to see Gaboff, and we talked about my regular job and how much medical terminology I knew. He then went on to explain that since the company was local and there were only about thirty-five Negro doctors in town, it would only be a part-time job for which I seemed perfectly suited. It was necessary to see each doctor only once every two to three months. He described what I was expected to do and took me out on several calls to introduce me and hear him talk to the doctors. After that I was to go out on my own to make the office detail calls.

The doctors' office hours were staggered throughout the day and into early evening. They would begin as early as 8:00 a.m., the latest hours being from 7:00 to 9:00 p.m. Calls by detail men during the evening hours were not looked upon kindly by the doctors. It took some maneuvering on my part to be able to make calls, but inasmuch as Dr. Blalock had more or less given the go-ahead for me to subsidize my salary by some means, I had wasted no time. Within two weeks, I was ready to begin making office calls.

Fortunately, our research was of a chronic nature and the experimental surgical procedure could be scheduled, as opposed to acute experiments, which would have required my presence in the laboratory throughout the day. I kept the bag containing medical samples and literature in the trunk of my car. By modifying my work schedule and lunch break, I was able to call on most of the Negro doctors in Baltimore in less than three months.

One of the company's products was a widely used antacid, an aluminum hydroxide gel that was superior to any product then on the market because it had no constipating side effects. The gel was also being dispensed by the Johns Hopkins pharmacy, which was never mentioned in doing a detail. Most doctors were prescribing a similar but less-desirable product of a large national drug company. About six months after I began making rounds, another Negro "detail man" appeared in Baltimore, representing a competitor. Gaboff knew of his presence before I did and told me of it, saying that I must be hurting the competitor's business. After that time, Negroes representing several of the larger national drug and pharmaceutical houses began to appear in the offices of Negro doctors in Baltimore.

I never used the name of Hopkins when I visited doctors' offices because I preferred that they not know of my association for several reasons. Whether true or not, Hopkins had a city-wide reputation of having the lowest-paying jobs in town for Negroes; I was probably trying to change that image. Few laymen knew me and those who did only knew that I worked for Hopkins, but not in what capacity. Our neighbors wondered how it happened that my wife didn't work and I worked for Hopkins. Another reason was that as a full-time detail man out on the street trying to make a go of it, I anticipated more cooperation from doctors wanting a Negro to succeed in this field, which previously had been closed to us. The doctors treated me well after they recovered from the initial shock of seeing a Negro detail man. The initial call usually took about an hour, which was more time than doctors usually allowed for a patient, and more time than was allowed for any detail man.

These regular office-hour calls were not by appointment. The detail man went into the doctor's waiting room, sat, and waited his turn. A composite of an initial visit would be as follows: I enter the waiting room, where two patients are seated. I sit down and put my bag under the chair. Expecting to wait almost an hour, I pick up a magazine and begin reading. The doctor calls one patient, then another. At last it is my turn. The doctor comes out of his office, so I stand with my bag in hand. The doctor sees the bag, then in one breath says, "Man, I don't want to buy anything.

Who are you? What do you have in that bag?" I reply only to the last question, telling him I have professional samples, literature, and information for him. He lets me into his office, and I introduce myself and the company I represent. Saying he never heard of the company, he offers me a seat. Opening my bag, I begin talking and get out a sample and brochure, which I pass to him. He asks a few questions about the product and the company. Then he asks if I'm a pharmacist. When I say no, he wants to know how I learned medical terminology. Had I flunked out of medical school? I tell him no and explain that I worked in a medical research laboratory for about fifteen years. Then he wants to know where. I tell him Nashville, for about eleven years, then about five years here. Where did you work here? Hopkins. What kind of laboratory were you in? Surgical research. Surgical research, he repeats. A quizzical expression comes over his face as he asks my name. I repeat it. Oh, yes, he recognizes the name and remembers having heard of me in connection with Dr. Blalock and the Blue Baby operation. Then a long discussion follows. He wants to know what part I played, and if what he heard was true. The next question is why I quit Hopkins. I had not quit Hopkins. If I still worked for them, why would I be doing this on the side? Couldn't Hopkins pay me for what I did? So why not quit and do this full time?

Often they would say that Dr. Blalock should pay me out of his own pocket with all the money he's making from that operation. I explained that Dr. Blalock was on a salary the same as I—a much larger salary, but still a salary. Numerous doctors said they would prescribe products to help me, but two of them bluntly stated that I was crazy. I also heard expressions such as "You're being made a fool of"; "if they want your services, let them pay you"; "you're subsidizing Hopkins, not yourself, work for them, but get your money from someone else"; and "Hopkins is making money as a result of work you've done—they have the money to pay you." The remarks I heard in the first two or three weeks of making detail calls on the Negro doctors in Baltimore only bolstered my determination to leave Hopkins.

Several weeks after the agreement with Dr. Blalock and the university had been reached, I told Gaboff that I could no longer continue the detail calls, saying that I just didn't have the time. He wasn't aware that my salary at Hopkins had been a problem and that I had been planning to leave town, or that Dr. Blalock had been negotiating in an effort to keep me there. Gaboff offered me a full-time job with the company, planning to expand the territory to cover Washington, D.C., York, Pa., and as far east as Wilmington, Del. I told him I had an 18-month commitment to Hopkins and could not accept the offer, which was better than the one I'd accepted from Hopkins. Even so, I could not be sure of long-term security, and detailing wasn't nearly as interesting as research. To entice me into continuing the part-time detail, Gaboff offered another increase in the per-call pay. I continued to make calls for over a year, but at a slower pace than that of the first six or eight weeks.

Dr. Blalock had said he didn't necessarily want to know about other employment, so I never told him about the Ralph Winton Company. The venture was a success in several ways. First, my per-call pay was increased after only two weeks. I could only assume that the Negro doctors had responded to my presence and that it was paying off for the company. Second, a new field of employment had been opened for Negroes in Baltimore as representatives of many of the nationally known drug and pharmaceutical houses.

A high percentage of the surgical staff had gone into military service with the Hopkins Medical Unit soon after the United States entered World War II. The few that remained had to cover the duties and responsibilities of all. With teaching and clinical duties, little time was left for research. Even the number of interns and house staff officers was reduced by the military. For the little research being done other than our own, Dr. Blalock let things stand without an M.D. directing the laboratory after Dr. Edgar Poth left the institution in mid-1942. As Dr. Thomas B. Turner tells it, "At Vanderbilt, Thomas assisted Blalock in his studies on shock and later in the investigations of renal blood flow in relation to hypertension. By the time they moved to Baltimore, Thomas had become an accomplished animal surgeon and was able to perform alone many intricate surgical procedures. His presence assured that Blalock's studies could continue virtually without interruption. As the younger surgeons went off to war one by one, Thomas became the de facto director of the Hunterian surgical laboratories and a key instructor in the ever popular student course in animal surgery."[17]

There was no central employment office at the Medical School. Within months after Poth's departure, I was taking care of our personnel. Adolph Stoll was drafted into the armed services and had to be replaced. I was handling the purchase of necessary surgical and laboratory supplies and equipment, chemicals, and drugs. There was no central purchasing at the Medical School, thus it was necessary to ascertain what vendors supplied needed supplies and material. Tom Satterfield was of tremendous help in that he had been on the job a long time and knew the representatives of most companies that furnished laboratory supplies. He was also familiar with the purchasing procedure. Louis Miller, a well-known figure around Johns Hopkins, represented Baltimore's largest surgical and hospital supply company. Lou Miller had begun making deliveries after school hours for Murray-Baumgarter, bicycling to hospitals and doctor's offices. As a representative of the company in his adult years, he made regular rounds of the hospital and medical school. Beside the information he carried in his briefcase, he had a wealth of knowledge on almost every item comprising laboratory and hospital supplies. A tall, pleasant, friendly, conscientious businessman, he gave me the liberty to call him whenever I had a question. Being new in the field of purchasing, I took advantage of his offer. Although my need may have been unrelated to his line of supplies, he never hesitated to get the information. When Dr. Blalock had asked to have something made, such as the Blalock clamp, Lou Miller was the first name that came to mind; thus Murray-Baumgarter made the clamp. Miller, who became president of the company, retired several years ago.

Mr. Burgan, Business Manager of the School of Medicine, procured dogs for all departments. Once the dogs were drawn from his supply, they became departmental responsibility. At this point, I was responsible for procurement of their feed, bedding, disinfectants, other supplies, and the personnel needed to care for them seven days a week, all holidays included. I was also responsible for maintenance of the laboratory equipment and facilities. Essentially, it was a matter of keeping the laboratory functional and functioning for student classes in operative (dog) surgery, Blalock research, and what few others were doing research at that time.

In late 1945, surgical staff members began returning to their posts and new doctors were being added to the staff; thus there was an immediate upswing in the amount of research being done in the laboratory. This, in turn, increased the amount of required technical help, materials, supplies, and equipment. This increase had been so gradual that I was able to keep pace with growing administrative responsibility. Even though I was taking paper work home, I didn't complain to Dr. Blalock.

Purchasing was done directly from the vendor, and invoices were sent to me in the laboratory. I would initial them and send them to Dr. Blalock's office, where they would be recorded, coded, and forwarded to the Homewood campus for payment. In late 1946 or early 1947, Hanlon was appointed director of the laboratory and I was instructed to send the invoices to him. When he received the first batch he called me to his office. He wanted a breakdown of each invoice, whom the material was for, on what project it was to be used, and if the prices were competitive—in essence, justification. After we'd gone over each item, I said I was happy he was taking over and that I would direct all requests to him or to his office. This he flatly refused, telling me to continue what I was doing because it was easier for me, since I knew the routine of where and how to get things. I agreed to do so with the stipulation that there would be no accounting that had not been required previously. I explained that this was all being done above and beyond my responsibility for Dr. Blalock's research program.

I had learned the routine the hard way and it was now relatively easy, as I had "grown" with the amount of activity in the laboratory over the past few years. My acceptance of the responsibility from Hanlon seemingly precluded any attempt at take-over by any of his numerous official successors as director of the laboratory. Had I realized the future headaches in store, I don't think I would have gone along with him so easily. The amount of work and responsibility was still on the increase, with no decrease in the Professor's research program. I already had a clipboard on my desk marked "Your Wants and Needs." When I was busy with research, people were referred to it to write their requests.

I cannot recall that Tom Satterfield had ever complained of illness or lost a day from the laboratory because of it. However, he began to complain of back pain in fall 1947. Hopkins doctors examined him and gave him medication to alleviate the pain, but he had no relief. More examinations, X-rays, and laboratory tests revealed nothing, so he was given more medication and told to get a corset and lose weight. The pain only became worse as time passed. Shortly after Christmas, he was having excruciating pain; then one day at the urinal in the laboratory he noticed that his urine was not normal in color. He called this to the attention of his doctor; further tests and X-rays showed that Tom had an enlarged kidney. Surgery revealed not only an enormous tumorous kidney, but also numerous metastatic tumors.

I had never had such an experience and had not realized how close Tom and I had become. During his illness, he insisted that I shave him three times a week. If I didn't visit him the other four days, he wanted to know why. As his condition deteriorated, he pleaded that I knew all the people around Hopkins and surely could get someone to help him. He was in constant pain, and I'm not sure he realized what was wrong with him. During his last seven to ten days, he was so heavily sedated that I don't think he knew I was keeping him shaved. Seeing him in that condition, I was relieved but saddened when he died on March 15, 1948. I had often asked for Tom's advice on running the laboratory as well as on research problems. I had trusted his judgment and on receiving it would often tell him he was a gentleman and a scholar. I was very surprised to learn that he had only gone through the eighth grade at St. Matthews Parish School, which was located on Washington Street across from the medical school. Indeed, I had lost a very good friend and co-worker.

With Tom's passing, I had to replace him, which, because of his years of experience, would be virtually impossible. Finding a dependable, intelligent, responsible individual to fill the position would be no easy task. Dr. Hanlon and I had numerous interviews, but only one applicant impressed us. This fifty-eight-year-old candidate had been a domestic helper and chauffeur for years, but the family he'd worked for had died out and he was unemployed. Dr. Hanlon and I were confident in his intelligence, ability, dependability, and learning capability. However, if we trained him in a field with which he wasn't familiar, how many years of service could we reasonably expect? Despite our concern, we made the right decision and hired Claude Brown, who proved to be everything we'd hoped for. He quickly learned his duties and was of tremendous help to me for much longer than Dr. Hanlon and I had projected. He took care of the general overseeing of the laboratory and saw that the experimental operating room ran smoothly by informing me when supplies were low or problems arose.

One of Claude's favorite researchers was Dr. Amos Koontz, who had been a colonel in the Hopkins Medical Unit and commanding officer of the Eighteenth General Hospital during World War II. Dr. Koontz, a private practitioner specializing in hernia repair, had set aside one morning a week to work in the laboratory. Many new materials, mainly plastics, were coming onto the market, and they included sutures, meshes, and woven materials. Dr. Koontz tested many of these on laboratory animals for possible use in hernia repair in humans. Dr. Koontz was strictly an army man, timing and prescribing the way things should be done. This exacting physician who had given tongue-lashings to several laboratory personnel got along perfectly with Claude Brown.

13

Having completed his internship, Thomas N. P. Johns returned to the laboratory as William S. Halsted Fellow of 1947–48. The development of a technique for the production of an interatrial septal defect as a possible method of treatment of transposition of the great vessels had occurred during the year of his absence. We continued, however, to attempt to produce transposition, still without success.

One of his major efforts was in relation to the treatment of mitral-valve insufficiency, for which no satisfactory method of treatment had been developed. Usually caused by rheumatic inflammation of the mitral valve, leaflets become thickened and scarred. The chordae tendinae become involved and there is sufficient loss of motion to prevent the valve leaflets from approximating properly during systole. The edges of the leaflets are irregular and there is no standard contour shape or form to the orifice in the condition. Johns set out to make a prosthesis that would be mobile and at the same time conform to whatever shape or contour the valve's edges might have. He tried several materials—inverted vein or pericardial sacs filled with blood and blood-filled sacs made of plastic film—none of which worked satisfactorily.

Using a piece of polyvinyl sponge (Ivalon), he fashioned a prosthesis with an elliptical body with cylindrical extensions on each end for anchoring. The elliptical portion of the prosthesis was suspended between the commissures parallel to the apposing edges of the mitral valve leaflets (see figs. 38, 39, 40). The results were quite satisfactory, and the prostheses were well tolerated. Autopsies revealed that they had been properly placed and were still mobile. The prostheses were covered with endothelium with no thrombi attached.[43] This was one of many steps taken before artificial circulation made open-heart procedures possible under direct vision. After completing his surgical residency in 1952, Dr. Johns went to the Medical College of Virginia as Assistant Professor of Surgery in 1953 and is currently in private practice in Richmond.

There was, and still is, much interest in and emphasis on coronary heart disease. Many investigators were at work in the attempt to increase the blood supply to the myocardium. We were evaluating the procedure of Dr. Claude Beck, of Cleveland, who attempted to increase the circulation in the myocardium by reversing the coronary blood flow through the coronary sinus. If this could be accomplished, blood could be supplied to

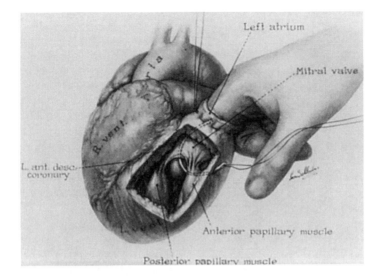

Fig. 38. Correction of mitral insufficiency. Before the perfection of extracorporeal circulation—the heart-lung machine—numerous attempts were made to surgically treat many congenital and acquired diseases of the heart by so-called "blind" operations, in which the surgeon identified structures by digital examination. In the procedure used by Thomas N. P. Johns, a polyvinyl sponge prosthesis closes the gap between the diseased valve cusps during systole. Sutures of heavy silk are passed through the wall of the ventricle through the orifice of the mitral valve and out of the opening in the left atrium. From Johns, T. N. P., and Blalock, A.: Mitral insufficiency, Annals of Surgery *140:335, September 1954, with permission.*

an undernourished area of the myocardium distal to the point of a coronary artery occlusion. Most of the experiments were performed by anastomosing the proximal end of the divided right carotid artery to the coronary sinus at or near its orifice in the right atrium. In some experiments the sinus was ligated, in others it was left patent. To evaluate any possible protection the procedure might give against a coronary occlusion, we ligated a coronary artery. A large series of experiments was performed with several variations, but the results were inconclusive.[44]

Dr. Marshal C. Sanford, who worked with Dr. Johns on this project, had received his M.D. degree from the Medical School in 1942 and had interned in surgery in the hospital. He received part of his resident training overseas with the Hopkins Medical Unit. Returning to Hopkins, he completed his residency in 1948. In appearance, he personified the "man of distinction," a picture used to advertise a brand-name whiskey of that time, and for this he good-naturedly took more than his share of kidding. He was briefly on the full-time staff before going into surgical practice

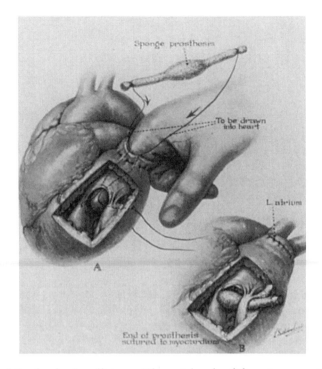

Fig. 39.   Mitral valve insufficiency. The atrial ends of the sutures are tied to the polyvinyl sponge prosthesis. As traction is made on the ventricular ends of the sutures, the sponge is pulled into the ventricle. Its ends emerge through the epicardial surface and are sutured in place. From Johns, T. N. P., and Blalock, A.: Mitral insufficiency, Annals of Surgery *140:335, September 1954, with permission.*

first in Washington, D.C., then in Fort Lauderdale, Fla. He is currently a gentleman farmer on his Coosaw Plantation near Dale, S.C.

While working on the problem of coronary heart disease, we performed some experiments in which we found it was technically possible to use an arterial graft between the aorta and the coronary artery to supply blood to the myocardium. To accomplish this, we perfused the coronary artery by using a short segment of small polyethylene tubing placed within the coronary artery and tied to isolate and bypass the site of the anastomosis. On completion of anastomosis, the segment of tubing was removed through a small incision made between previously placed sutures. The mortality rate was prohibitively high, the procedure having been performed without the heart-lung machine, which hadn't been developed. Thus the effort was abandoned, and the results were not reported.

Dr. Raymond O. Heimbecker of Toronto, a Fellow of the National Research Council of Canada in 1949–50, had come to work in Dr.

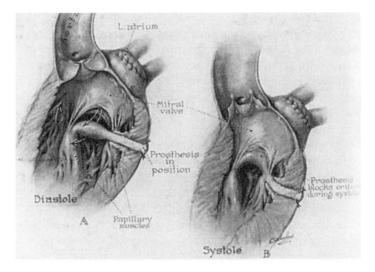

Fig. 40. *Mitral valve insufficiency, intended motion of prosthesis. In diastole the prosthesis does not obstruct the inflow tract; in systole the valve leaflets close against it. Direction of blood flow indicated by arrows. From Johns, T. N. P., and Blalock, A.: Mitral insufficiency,* Annals of Surgery, *140:335, September 1954, with permission.*

Blalock's laboratory. Dr. Blalock had for years been interested in the reversal of circulation. My first assignment on arriving at Hopkins in 1941 was to attempt reversal of circulation of the blood in a segment of small intestine. The results were negative and not reported. In 1948 Johns and I had attempted reversal of the flow of blood in the myocardium. In these experiments, there was no method available to determine if and how much reverse flow had been produced or how much blood was simply shunted into the right atrium through the thebesian veins. In the interim between these two studies, Dr. Blalock had had me attempt reversal of the flow of blood in the pelvis and posterior extremities. This had been accomplished by sectioning the aorta and inferior cava near their termini and anastomosing the proximal end of the aorta to the distal end of the cava and the proximal end of the cava to the distal end of the aorta. None of these animals survived over twenty-four hours, and none showed an obvious cause of death. I had also attempted reversal of the flow of blood in a single posterior extremity and in a lobe of lung. None of the above experiments were satisfactory or conclusive, and the results of our work and that of other investigators had been difficult to evaluate and interpret.

In an effort to determine if it was indeed physiologically possible to reverse the flow of blood through the capillaries, Dr. Blalock had Heimbecker and me perform experiments in which direct observations, using a binocular microscope, were made of the flow of blood through the capillaries. To document our observations, we used a Kodak movie camera to take photographs through the microscope.

The observations were done mostly on cats that had been anesthetized with Nembutal intraperitoneally. The vessels in the intestinal mesentery were found to be the most satisfactory for the study. We made a small, low, midline incision through which the terminal ileum was delivered, which then exposed the mesenteric blood vessels to this area. The vessels were followed to the base of the mesentery, and large branches of the mesenteric artery and vein were prepared for cannulation. The femoral artery and vein were similarly prepared. The animals were heparinized. The cannulae were of polyethylene tubing of a suitable size. Short segments of polyethlyene tubing of an intermediate size were used to adapt the smaller (mesenteric) cannula to the larger (femoral) cannula. A heavy ligature was placed around the end of the segment of intestine to be isolated, including the connecting mesenteric vessels, thus effectively occluding collateral circulation (see fig. 41). A quartz rod and a 500-watt light source were used to illuminate the point of observation. The field was kept moist with a gentle flow of warm Ringer's solution. In addition to the observations on the direction of blood-flow, the rate of flow through the isolated segment was determined by temporarily disconnecting the venous cannula and timing the flow of blood. Oxygen consumption of the segment of intestine was calculated by using the arteriovenous oxygen differences of the blood.

With the cannulae in place, studies were made with the flow of blood in the normal direction, femoral artery to mesenteric artery, through the capillaries and returning mesenteric vein to femoral vein. Reversal of flow was then produced by attaching the inflow arterial (femoral) cannula to the mesenteric vein and the outflow mesenteric artery to the femoral vein. Thus, the capillary bed of the area was observed with the blood-flow in normal and reverse directions. These observations were demonstrated in motion pictures. Failure of the flow to reverse was usually due to incomplete occlusion of collateral arterial blood supply to the segment. The longest period the reversal of the circulation was observed was fifty-seven minutes.

It was interesting to observe the red blood cells tumble along edge over edge or roll along through a capillary as a coin will roll when dropped to the floor. The rate of flow of blood and the oxygen consumption of the segment of intestine were determined in ten experiments, which showed that acute reversal of the flow through the capillaries will occur if arterial blood at or near systemic arterial pressure is supplied on the venous end of the capillaries and is allowed to flow away on the arterial end of the capillary. It was also shown that the blood flowing in the reverse direction gives up oxygen to the tissues.[45]

Observation through a microscope of a field that was fluid made motion a problem. We were appalled by the motion set off in the field of observation when streetcars crossed intersecting tracks; they ran on Monument and Wolfe streets, which bordered the south and west sides of the block in which the Hunterian Laboratory was located. None of the four streets that bordered the block was smooth, and vibrations from large trucks set off excessive and intolerable motion. After 7 p.m. the volume of streetcar and truck traffic was reduced and we found it to our advantage to begin the experiments at this time. Even though we were performing these experiments at night, Dr. Blalock expected my daytime schedule to go on. We compromised, after some discussion, by my agreeing to come in at noon on the days following one of these experiments, which were never finished before midnight.

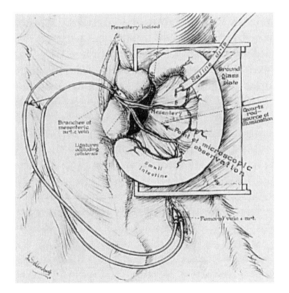

Fig. 41. The experimental procedure for the microscopic observation of the reversal of capillary blood flow. A segment of the intestine is delivered through an abdominal incision. A mesenteric artery and vein have been isolated. These vessels are connected by cannulae of plastic tubing to the femoral artery and vein. Braided silk occlude the intestine and collateral blood vessels. Arrow indicates points of microscopic observation. From Heimbecker, R.; Thomas, V.; and Blalock, A.: Experimental reversal of capillary blood flow, Circulation 4:116, July 1951, with permission of the American Heart Association, Inc.

Unaware that my name hadn't been offered in the publication of Dr. Blalock's scientific papers, which spanned the twenty years I'd worked with him, Dr. Heimbecker submitted a draft of this paper, naming as co-authors Dr. Blalock, himself, and me. Heimbecker, now Professor of Surgery at University of Western Ontario and Chief of Cardiovascular and Thoracic Surgery at University Hospital in London, Ontario, Canada, thought my contribution to the project warranted the inclusion of my name. To my knowledge, none of Dr. Blalock's numerous co-authors of laboratory reports had ever acted or thought along this line. The Professor, for whatever reason, did not remove it; as a result, this was the first paper on which my name appeared as co-author with that of Alfred Blalock, M.D.[45]

There was, and still is, an ongoing campaign by antivivisection groups to ban the use of dogs for research. In 1949 these groups became so powerful in Baltimore that the supply of dogs to our laboratory from the city pound was cut off. The supply of dogs being bought out of state was also threatened, with the arrests of men making deliveries to us. The University of Maryland School of Medicine, facing the same difficulty, joined us in bringing the matter to the attention of City Council. A hearing was held with both sides well represented, the antivivisectionists armed with numbers and loud voices, spokesmen for the medical institutions armed with irrefutable facts. Speaking at the hearing, among others, were Dr. Alan M. Chesney, Dean of the School of Medicine of Johns Hopkins, and Mr. Russel Brock (later Lord Brock), then Visiting Professor of Surgery from Guy's Hospital in London. They gave running accounts of the progress in medical science through the use of dogs, citing the work of Dr. Halsted on intestinal surgery. When Dean Chesney, a mild-mannered and soft-spoken man, rose to speak his voice was all but drowned out by the screams and cat-calls of the antivivisectionists. This seemed to be the only type of rebuttal they had to offer. The Blue Baby operation that recently had been developed at Hopkins was fresh in the minds of everyone in Baltimore. Although Dr. Blalock was out of town, Dr. Warfield Firor, Professor of Surgery at Hopkins, presented one of the little patients on whom the operation had been performed and was loudly booed.

City Council decided that the medical institutions could use some of the stray and unclaimed dogs from the Baltimore pound. The antivivisectionists would not accept that decision and secured enough signatures to bring the matter to referendum. Then the two daily newspapers joined the fray. One newspaper took the viewpoint of the antivivisectionists. The *Sunpapers*, siding with the medical institutions, sounded the cry to keep Baltimore one of the world's great medical centers, a reputation earned through research. Through editorials and articles, they informed the general public of specific developments and advancements made in the field of medicine through research. The question was on the ballot in the upcoming election, and on election day, medical students were on the streets near all polling places passing out literature. The antivivisectionists were soundly defeated by more than four to one.

During 1950 the Professor would be performing the one-thousandth Blue Baby operation, and there was general agreement that something should be done to commemorate the occasion. Dr. Hanlon suggested having Yousef Karsh, the noted Canadian portrait photographer, take one of his famous pictures of Dr. Blalock. The idea was attractive, but everyone knew that the Professor, who was modest about publicity, would not easily be persuaded to sit through what to him would be an ordeal. Dr. Ravitch contacted Karsh, and accepting the pretext that the picture was to be used in Karsh's proposed book on notable figures in medicine, Dr. Blalock consented. As it turned out, Karsh subsequently published a book on notable people in all walks of life, entitled *Portraits of Greatness*. Among the great, such as Winston Churchill, were five men of medicine, including Alfred Blalock. Karsh liked to know his subject's personality, which he would capture in his photographs. Karsh accompanied the Professor for two days, camera in hand. There were both formal and informal picture-taking sessions with outstanding results. On the second day, the Professor, remembering that this picture was to appear in Great Men of Medicine, told Karsh that if he were interested in doctors and medicine, he should see the Blue Baby operation being performed. Karsh accepted the invitation and was awed by the Professor's performance.

Almost unbelievably, Ravitch received the photographic proofs on the day the one-thousandth Blue Baby operation was performed. Ravitch immediately telephoned everyone in town who had been on any of the Blue Baby surgical teams. Each was instructed to bring a bottle of scotch or bourbon to the Professor's house to celebrate at a given hour that evening. Miss Olive Berger, who had administered anesthesia to the vast majority of the Blue Babies, was also called. The doctors and their wives converged almost simultaneously on the Blalock residence on Underwood Road at the appointed time. Mrs. Blalock had been forewarned and being the marvelous hostess she was, had prepared for them. After socializing for a while, the nineteen photographic proofs were spread out on the living-room floor and passed around. Mrs. Blalock selected her favorite shot (fig. 42), which was difficult since several seemed just as good. Then the Professor sat in his wing chair and assumed a role that few had seen before and were not likely to see again. Aside from his immediate family, he was surrounded by his closest friends; thus he was happy and perfectly relaxed. He began speaking in a manner that was informal, warm and

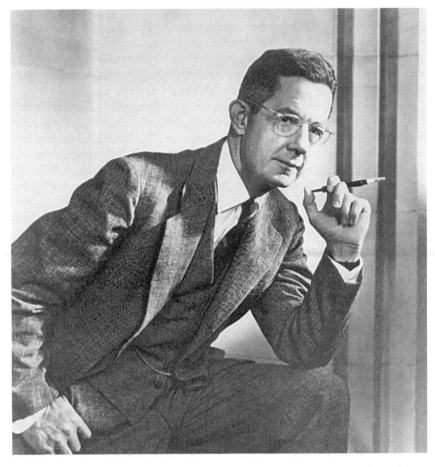

Fig. 42.   The official Blue Baby portrait of Alfred Blalock, by Yousef Karsh.

friendly, lucid, and all-encompassing as everyone sat almost spellbound on chairs or on the floor around him. When he finished he rose and said he was going upstairs. Most of those present thought it had been one of the most delightful and memorable evenings they had ever experienced.

The medical students generally enjoyed working around the laboratory and assisting in the experimental surgical procedures. In late 1950, J. Alex Haller, then a medical student, was assisting in a procedure being performed by James Isaacs, M.D., an assistant resident. The procedure was taking much longer than had been anticipated. After two hours or more had elapsed, Isaacs suggested that maybe I should start some intravenous fluid. While preparing the fluid I noticed that Haller was a little pale, as if he was the one who needed the fluid. I tugged at Haller's pant leg and asked in which leg he preferred I give the fluid, which made everyone laugh.

Haller received his M.D. degree in 1951. He completed his surgical residency in 1959, having spent two of those years in study and training in Zurich. He remained on the full-time staff at Hopkins, but during his early years often found himself with insufficient funds for the research he wanted to carry on in the laboratory. It was my responsibility to keep everyone busy who wanted to work. With the leverage I had in the expenditure of funds for research, I did not find it too difficult to keep him happy. By allowing him to use supplies from stock, which were paid for with other funds, and by using funds from large grants to purchase items he needed, I helped him keep a continuous research program going. One of his most significant projects was intrauterine surgery, in which he produced congenital defects in the fetus of sheep.[46] The congenital defects thus produced were studied and surgically treated in the young lambs. Haller is Robert Garrett Professor of Pediatric Surgery at Johns Hopkins.

Jerry Harris came to the Surgical Research Laboratory in 1966. Working with Dr. Alex Haller, he became a very efficient and conscientious surgical research technician. His diligent efforts were very important to the successful completion of Dr. Haller's research on the production of congenital defects in the fetus of sheep. Harris assisted in teaching the techniques to incoming Fellows and performed many of the Caesarian sections, keeping the newborn lambs alive. The survival of these lambs was all important to future study and the development of corrective procedures on the defects previously produced.

14

Dr. Jerome H. Kay, a graduate of the University of California at San Francisco, came to work in the laboratory as of July 1, 1950. He already had four or five years of post-doctoral (surgical house staff) training in Dallas under Dr. Carl Moyer. He began working with me on a cardiac project that was in progress, but Dr. Blalock wanted him to have a project of his own. He wanted the Fellows to have ideas and interests that they would like to investigate, some question to which they would like to find the answer. Dr. Blalock considered this a year during their training when they could read, think, study, and work. No other year of training would offer these combined opportunities.

Cardiac arrest may occur in any type of surgery under anesthesia. Considering the amount of cardiac surgery that was being performed at Hopkins and elsewhere and the relatively high incidence of cardiac arrest then occurring in those cases, Dr. Kay began to read about the subject. Cardiac arrest may occur in either of two forms: (1) ventricular standstill in which there is little or no contraction of the muscle fibers or (2) ventricular fibrillation in which there is uncoordinated contraction or twitching of the muscle fibers. He found that clinical cases of successful resuscitation had been reported. The earliest report was in 1947 by Dr. Claude Beck of Western Reserve University at Cleveland, Ohio. Numerous investigators had done research on the problem, for which there were two existing approaches: (1) the use of electric shock and (2) the use of drugs or cardiac stimulants. No one seemed to have an organized plan of attack. With various methods being used and advocated, Dr. Kay set out to determine the most satisfactory procedure for restoring an effective heart beat.

In searching through the literature, Dr. Kay came upon the name of William B. Kouwenhoven. While discussing cardiac arrest with Dr. Blalock, Dr. Kay asked if he knew Kouwenhoven. Dr. Blalock thought that Kouwenhoven had been a professor of electrical engineering at the University but was probably retired. Kay followed up the lead and found that Dr. Kouwenhoven was still on the Homewood campus as Dean of the School of Engineering and Professor and Chairman of Electrical Engineering. Dr. Kouwenhoven, Dr. Orthello Langworthy, and Dr. Donald Hooker had done research on defibrillation of the heart by the use of an electric current in the 1920s and early 1930s. They had confirmed the findings of Prevost and Batelli in 1899, that ventricular fibrillation could be arrested by electric shock.

Dr. Kay had Dr. Kouwenhoven make an apparatus for him that would deliver a 130-volt, 60-cycle electric current. For the experiments, the apparatus was more or less an assembly of parts on a wooden table. The parts were a Variac transformer to regulate the voltage of the current, a foot switch, a pair of electrodes, and a convenience outlet into which the electrodes were plugged. The electrodes were brass disks 1 inch in diameter with handles of ¼-inch brass rod, 9 inches long. The handles were insulated by rubber tubing with ⅛-inch walls.

The experiments were performed on dogs, using positive-pressure ether anesthesia. The heart was exposed through the left fifth interspace and the pericardium was opened. Blood pressure and/or electrocardiogram (EKG) was recorded. A 30-volt, 60-cycle electric current was used to produce fibrillation of the heart. Upon beginning to massage the heart, Dr. Kay realized that cardiac massage was not just a matter of squeezing the heart. To achieve effective cardiac massage—that is, force blood through the coronary arteries and circulate it throughout the body—the position of the hand on the heart and the vigor of the massage were of great importance (see fig. 43). The heart was firmly and deliberately squeezed 40 to 50 times per minute. This rate, although seemingly slow as compared to the normal heart rate, allowed adequate time for the heart chambers to refill with blood before the next massage. By this method, systemic blood pressures of from 80 to 150 millimeters of mercury were obtained in over 40 percent of the experiments.

After the heart was massaged for three minutes or more, the electrodes were applied—one beneath the right auricular appendage, the other on the left ventricle near the apex of the heart. Defibrillation would be attempted by an electric shock of 130-volt, 60-cycle current. When massage was begun immediately on production of fibrillation, subsequent defibrillation was easy. In order to make the ventricular fibrillation as well as the resultant ventricular standstill following defibrillation more difficult to treat, massage was delayed for from three to seven minutes in some of the experiments. The difficulties made it possible to test various cardiac stimulants.

Dr. Kay demonstrated to Dr. Blalock how he could fibrillate the heart, massage it for as long as an hour, and then defibrillate it.[47] The test animals would walk around the next day, showing no neurological signs. Dr. Blalock had Drs. Kay and Kouwenhoven make a defibrillator unit that could be used in the general operating rooms. I assembled the unit in the laboratory under Dr. Kouwenhoven's supervision (see fig. 44). After Dr. Kay had tested it on animals, it was sent to the general operating

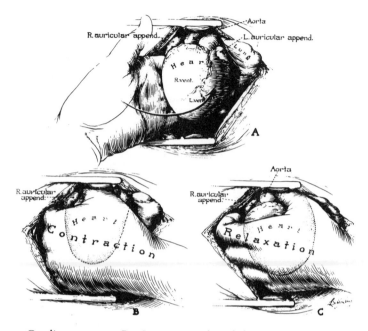

Fig. 43.   Cardiac massage. Dr. Jerome Kay found this position most effective in cardiac massage. In larger hearts, however, he found that it may be necessary to massage with one hand in front of the heart and the other in back. From Kay, J. H.: Treatment of cardiac arrest, Surgery, Gynecology & Obstetrics 93:682– 90, fig. 1, July 1951, with permission of Surgery, Gynecology & Obstetrics.

rooms.[48] When a patient went into cardiac arrest, Dr. Blalock would call Dr. Kay from the laboratory to the operating room to have him try to restart the heart. The procedure elicited interest at other institutions, and I assembled defibrillator units for the National Institute of Health, Baylor Hospital in Houston, the University of Washington, and others.

During the progress of these experiments, Dr. Kouwenhoven began coming to the laboratory at the request of Dr. Kay. For several months he spent two or three hours a week, and on one of these occasions Dr. Blalock met Dr. Kouwenhoven. The Professor, favorably impressed by Dr. Kouwenhoven's keen interest in and knowledge of cardiac arrest, invited him to work in the laboratory. Dr. Kouwenhoven, an electrical engineer, had always wondered about the effect of electric currents on the human body and was happy to cooperate with us in our studies. He had become involved in the problem of cardiac fibrillation as a result of an appeal by the electric power industry. In the mid-1920s, the power companies had become concerned about the increasing number of fatalities suffered by linemen. In 1928 Dr. Kouwenhoven joined a Hopkins team that was investigating the problem. Their goal was the resuscitation of these linemen.

Dr. Blalock assigned a laboratory in the old Hunterian building to Dr. Kouwenhoven, who brought in transformers, capacitors, switches, timers, and all sorts of electrical gear he'd accumulated on the Homewood campus. By this time, the studies on open-chest resuscitation were

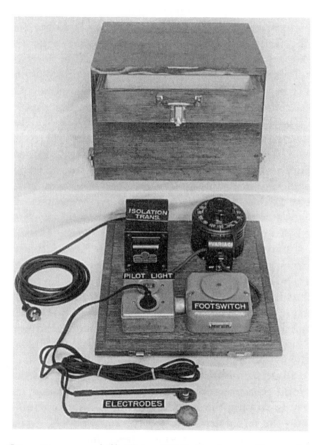

Fig. 44.   *Operating-room defibrillator. While Dr. Jerome Kay performed experiments on open-chest defibrillation of the heart, the apparatus was essentially a collection of parts on a wooden instrument table. Under the supervision of Dr. William B. Kouwenhoven, Dr. Kay and I built the above unit. From Kouwenhoven, W. B., and Kay, J. H.: A simple electrical apparatus for the clinical treatment of ventricular fibrillation,* Surgery *30:781, November 1951, with permission.*

about completed and a defibrillator unit was in the general operating rooms. Dr. Kay and I then set out to help Dr. Kouwenhoven in his attempt to reach his ultimate goal, external defibrillation of the heart.

Fortunately, the laboratory assigned to Dr. Kouwenhoven was on the top floor, away from the main stream of traffic in the building. In these closed-chest defibrillation experiments, electric currents as high as 4,000 volts were used. On the discharge of a capacitor at this voltage, the crackling sound, as of lightning, could be heard on the floor below.

It was always said as a joke but well understood that if thunder were ever heard—meaning the sound of someone falling to the floor—a person from the floor below was to bring an animal endotracheal tube posthaste. The recipient of the electric charge would be intubated and put on an animal respirator until help could be summoned from the hospital. We were just beginning the studies as related to external defibrillation, but we were confident we could successfully resuscitate a patient with an open chest. There was no doubt in my mind that the above "joke" would have been carried out if the unfortunate event occurred.

As in the experiments on the open-chest defibrillation of the heart, blood pressure and/or EKG were being monitored and/or recorded. When there was difficulty in defibrillating the heart, various stimulants would be injected by cardiac puncture. We were aware from open-chest studies that in the absence of an effective heart beat, these stimulants would remain in the heart chambers. However, on massage, the blood containing the cardiac stimulant would be forced out of the heart into the aorta and into the coronary vessels and thus affect the myocardium itself. In these experiments, however, the chest was not open. In order to massage the heart and thus force the blood and the stimulant into the aorta and coronary arteries, it was necessary to compress the chest wall against it. This was accomplished in two ways: (1) by intermittently compressing both sides of the chest simultaneously or (2) by applying intermittent pressure just above the xyphoid in some dogs with relatively flat chests. The experiments were all performed with the animals in a supine position. I do not recall the blood pressures obtained by these methods, but the methods were effective in forcing the blood containing the stimulants out of the heart and into the circulation and the coronary vessels, giving us a fair degree of success in the resuscitation of these animals. The animals were on a positive-pressure respirator, so no emphasis was placed on respirations. The project seemed to have been well under way when Dr. Kay's tenure as a Fellow ended almost abruptly.

Dr. Kay's first year had been so productive that the Professor asked him to stay for a second year. Although Dr. Kay thought he would spend his entire second year in the laboratory, an assistant resident was needed on the surgical house staff; thus Dr. Blalock called him into the Hospital to fill the position as of January 1952. Dr. Blalock also removed me from direct involvement with Dr. Kouwenhoven and the project. Some of the projects that Dr. Kay and I had been doing concurrently with the defibrillation projects had to be completed and numerous follow-up studies had to be done. With Dr. Kay gone, this became my full responsibility. Several years passed before much was heard of Dr. Kouwenhoven's project on external defibrillation of the heart. I must admit that at the time I did not fully appreciate how the development of a method for external defibrillation of the heart, aside from saving linemen's lives, would be of such tremendous and widespread benefit to the general public.

During the eighteen months Dr. Kay had been in the laboratory, our time had been rigidly scheduled. Besides the projects on open- and closed-chest defibrillation of the heart, there had been a never-ending series of experiments to produce, study, and correct models of both congenital and acquired abnormalities of the heart. After many years of work and experience, Dr. Kay and I were able to produce three of the abnormalities found in the tetralogy of Fallot. These were (1) the experimental production of a high interventricular septal defect, (2) the experimental production of pulmonary stenosis, and (3) right ventricular hypertrophy as a result of increased right ventricular pressure. We also produced insufficiency of the pulmonary valve.

Before Dr. Kay's arrival, I had made numerous attempts to produce an interventricular septal defect. The purpose was to study the chronic physiologic effects and possibly develop a method of closure. This had been done by introducing an instrument, a Halsted or Kelly hemostat, through a purse-string suture placed in the right ventricular wall. The tip of the instrument was then forced within the purse string through the ventricular wall and the interventricular septum into the left ventricle. The instrument was then opened slightly to spread the jaws and enlarge the hole made by the closed instrument. The instrument was withdrawn and the purse-string suture tied. The same approach to the septum was used employing a #11 knife blade. In our attempts, there had been no control of the size of the defect. If the defect was made too small, the animal would survive but the defect would subsequently close spontaneously. If the defect was too large, the animal would die within hours or a few days. In a discussion of the previous trials, Kay suggested that if we used a cork borer, removing a plug of the septal muscle, it might be possible to grade the size of the defect by using different sizes of borers, and that the defect, being round, might be less likely to close spontaneously. We tried the laboratory cork borers. The plug removed from the septum by the borer would not always be forced into the borer by the pressure in the ventricles. After losing the plug of septal muscle in the circulation on several occasions, Dr. Blalock suggested that we should put suction on the borer to retrieve the plug. Jones made a set of special borers from ³⁄₁₆ to ½ inch in diameter in ¹⁄₁₆-inch increments (see fig. 45).

The dogs were given positive-pressure ether anesthesia. The chest was opened through the left fourth interspace and the pericardium incised anterior to the left phrenic nerve. A mattress suture of silk was placed in the right ventricular muscle slightly below the origin of the pulmonary artery. A purse-string suture was placed around the mattress suture. With traction on the free ends of the mattress suture, an incision was made large enough to admit the tip of the left index finger. As the finger was withdrawn, the cork-borer cardiotome was inserted (see fig. 46). The purse string was then pulled tight around it to control bleeding. The tip of the instrument was advanced until it engaged the interventricular septum im-

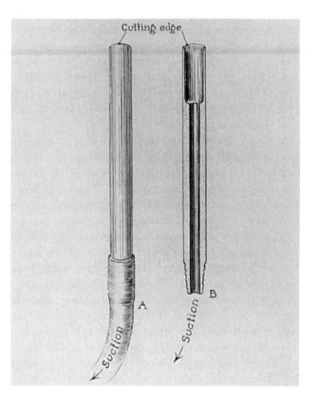

Fig. 45. *Diagram of the instrument used to produce an interventricular septal defect. A: Outside of instrument with rubber tubing leading to a suction apparatus. B: Sagittal section of instrument. From Kay, J. H.; Thomas, V. T.; and Blalock, A.: The experimental production of high interventricular septal defects,* Surgery, Gynecology & Obstetrics 96:529, May 1953, *with permission of* Surgery, Gynecology & Obstetrics.

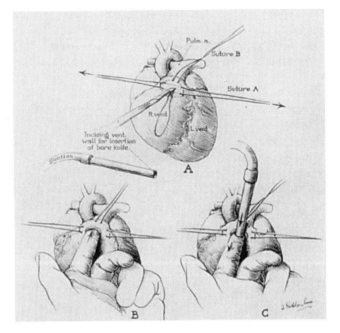

Fig. 46. *Method of production of an interventricular septal defect. A: Mattress and pursestring sutures have been placed immediately beneath the pulmonary valves and an incision is made into right ventricle while the mattress suture is held taut. B: The left index finger is inserted and the interventricular septum is palpated. C: The instrument is advanced as the finger is removed. From Kay, J. H.; Thomas, V. T.; and Blalock, A.: The experimental production of high interventricular septal defects,* Surgery, Gynecology & Obstetrics 96 : 529, May 1953, *with permission of* Surgery, Gynecology & Obstetrics.

mediately beneath the attachments of the pulmonary valve leaflets. At this point suction was applied; using a rotary motion, we advanced the cardiotome, trying to make it emerge directly beneath the attachment of the aortic valve in the left ventricle (see fig. 47). While still maintaining suction, we withdrew the instrument, and the previously placed mattress and purse-string sutures were tied. The plug of septal tissue that was removed usually was held inside the instrument by the suction.

The procedure was performed on 32 dogs and 19 survived for 48 days or more (see fig. 48). The survival rate varied directly with the size of the defect created. When the ½-inch-diameter cardiotome was used, three of four animals died of the physiological effects of the ventricular septal defect within 24 hours. The fourth was sacrificed at 2½ months with pronounced right-sided heart failure, ascites, and edema of the pos-

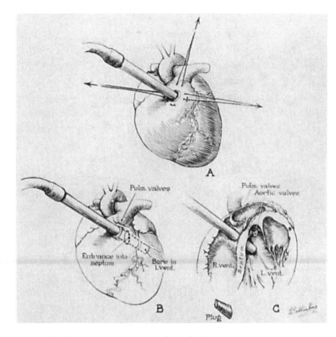

Fig. 47.   A: *As the instrument is introduced, the pursestring suture is pulled taut. B: The cardiotome is advanced until it engages the septum and the suction is turned on. C: With a rotary motion, the instrument is advanced through the septum. The cardiotome is withdrawn along with the plug of septum it contains. The left index finger is then placed into the right ventricle and dilates the defect. The finger is removed and the pursestring and mattress sutures are tied. The insert reveals the configuration of the plug of septal tissue that was removed. From Kay, J. H.; Thomas, V. T.; and Blalock, A.: The experimental production of high interventricular septal defects,* Surgery, Gynecology & Obstetrics 96:529, *May 1953, with permission of* Surgery, Gynecology & Obstetrics.

terior extremities. Using the $7/16$-inch-diameter cardiotome, all of three dogs died within 24 hours.

By using the $3/8$-inch-diameter cardiotome, we produced defects in 25 dogs, nine of which died in less than 14 days. The most common causes of death were congestive failure, hemorrhage from the site of the myocardial incision, and distemper. Three of the animals were sacrificed between the second and fifth months because there was no heart murmur. At autopsy, it was found that the defects had closed. All had been placed too far anteriorly and involved the wall of both the right and left ventricle.

Cardiac catheterizations were carried out on the remaining animals over a period of 7 to 13 months after the creation of the interventricular septal defects. Pressures were recorded and samples of blood for determination of oxygen content were collected from the right ventricle, the pulmonary artery, and the femoral artery. Total oxygen uptake was also determined. The results of these analyses were used to determine the right and left ventricular output of blood and the amount of blood that passed through the interventricular septal defect. Seven of the animals showed left-to-right-heart shunts that accounted for 30 to 49 percent of the pulmonary blood flow. All the animals showed some rise in the right ventricular pressure. Six had a right ventricular pressure of 50 millimeters of mercury or higher and one, a right ventricular pressure of 100 millimeters of mercury.

These defects were high in the septum, which is the most frequent anatomical position found clinically in congenital interventricular septal defects. The method was the only reported technique of producing interventricular septal defects that resembled congenital defects and remained patent over long periods of time.[49]

Numerous methods of producing pulmonary stenosis had been attempted. Dr. Kay and I were working so closely and intensely that our conversations seldom went beyond cardiac research problems. Neither of us recalls who presented the idea of using a strong irritant on the pulmonary valve cusps and sinus to produce scarring and fibrosis. We thought the reaction might be somewhat like the effect of rheumatic fever on the

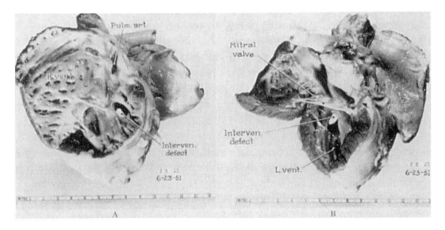

Fig. 48. Interventricular septal defect produced with the 9.3-mm. (³⁄₈-in.) instrument. Because of cardiac failure, the animal was sacrificed 78 days after production of defect. A: View of right ventricle showing the large patent defect beneath the pulmonary valves. B: View of left ventricle showing the large patent defect. From Kay, J. H.; Thomas, V. T.; and Blalock, A.: The experimental production of high interventricular septal defects, Surgery, Gynecology & Obstetrics *96:529, May 1953, with permission of* Surgery, Gynecology & Obstetrics.

valve leaflets producing dense scarring and fribrosis, thereby possibly constricting the pulmonary orifice.

A silver nitrate stick applied to the valve leaflets did not produce the desired scarring or damage in several animals on which it was used. Next, we tried several concentrations of a solution of sodium hydroxide, but even the application of a saturated solution of sodium hydroxide did not cause sufficient damage to produce the desired fibrous formation. Knowing that we were restricted in the length of time available for the irritant to damage the valves by the method we were using, almost in desperation, we decided to try concentrated (fuming) nitric acid, which should act in a matter of seconds.

The heart was approached through an incision in the left fourth interspace, with the dog under pressure ether anesthesia. The pericardium was incised anterior to the left phrenic nerve. Heavy braided silk ligatures were placed around the superior vena cava, the inferior vena cava, the azygos vein, and the pulmonary artery for temporary occlusion of the circulation (see fig. 49). Traction was put on all four ligatures, effectively blocking the flow of blood to the right ventricle except that from the coronary sinus. An incision was made in the pulmonary artery. The blood was aspirated from the right ventricle and pulmonary artery. The pulmonary valve cusps and the sinuses of Valsalva were painted with concentrated nitric acid (see fig. 50).

The traction on the four ligatures was released and a small amount of blood was allowed to flow through the incision in the pulmonary artery to flush out residual acid. Hemostats were placed at each end of the incision in the pulmonary artery and a straight Pott's clamp was applied to seal off the incision. The incision in the pulmonary artery was sutured with 5-0 silk and the Pott's clamp was removed. The circulation had been interrupted approximately 2½ minutes. After irrigation with copious amounts of saline solution, the pericardium and chest were closed with silk.

The procedure was performed on 29 dogs. Multiple cardiac catheterizations, for periods of from 2 to 19 months, demonstrated a pronounced increase in right ventricular pressure in all the animals thus treated, within 2 months.

Within 5 months 4 animals died of right-sided heart failure, 3 of these with ascites and edema of the lower abdomen and posterior extremities. Of the 29 dogs, 24 had right ventricular systolic pressures of 75 millimeters of mercury or higher; 11 of these had right ventricular pressures of 100 millimeters of mercury or higher. The lowest right ventricular pressure recorded was 50 millimeters of mercury; the highest was 140 millimeters of mercury. Pulmonary artery pressures remained essentially unchanged. In the 14 animals on which preoperative right ventricular

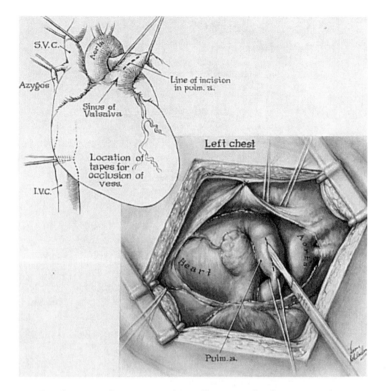

Fig. 49. *Production of stenosis and insufficiency of pulmonary valves. Approach to the pulmonary valves in the experimental production of pulmonic stenosis and of pulmonary insufficiency. The heart is exposed through an incision in the left fourth interspace. Temporary occluding ties are placed around the superior and inferior cavae, the azygos vein, and the distal portion of the main pulmonary artery. With traction made on all the temporary occluding ties, the pulmonary artery is opened longitudinally.* From Kay, J. H., and Thomas, V. T.: Experimental production of pulmonary stenosis, Archives of Surgery 69 : 651, November 1954, copyright 1954, American Medical Association, with permission.

pressures had been recorded, the highest pressure was 35 millimeters of mercury.

Autopsies revealed right ventricular hypertrophy. There was inelasticity of the proximal portion of the pulmonary artery with pronounced narrowing of the artery immediately distal to the insertion of the valve cusps. Most of the valve cusps had been destroyed.[50]

Pulmonary valvectomies were performed in order to study the chronic physiological and pathological effects of pulmonary insufficiency. The

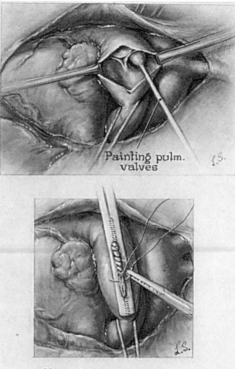

Fig. 50. Top: In the experimental production of pulmonary stenosis, the cusps and the sinuses of Valsalva are painted with concentrated nitric acid. Bottom: Closure of the incision in the pulmonary artery made to expose the valve cusps. Using mosquito forceps at each end of the incision, a straight Pott's clamp is applied for temporary closure of the incision. The incision is then closed with a continuous cardiovascular suture. Within two months, there is constriction of the outflow tract as demonstrated by an increase in the right ventricular pressure on cardiac catheterization. From Kay, J. H., and Thomas, V. T.: Experimental production of pulmonary stenosis, Archives of Surgery 69:651. November 1954, copyright 1954, American Medical Association, with permission.

method of approach to the pulmonary valve was the same as that used in the production of pulmonary stenosis. Under direct vision, the pulmonary valve cusps were excised (see fig. 51), and the incision in the pulmonary artery was closed.

Pulmonary insufficiency was produced in 15 dogs. One dog died of right-sided heart failure, with ascites and edema of the extremities, 8 months after the pulmonary valve was excised. A second animal stopped

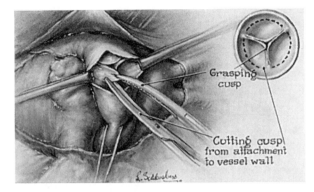

Fig. 51. Technique used in the experimental production of pulmonary insuffi-ciency. The valve cusps are completely excised. From Kay, J. H., and Thomas, V. T.: Experimental production of pulmonary insufficiency, Archives of Surgery 69:646, November 1954, copyright 1954, American Medical Association, with permission.

eating and died of inanition at 10 months after production of pulmonary insufficiency. In 10 of the 15 animals, the right ventricular pressure was 50 millimeters of mercury or higher; in 3 of these the systolic pressure was 90 millimeters of mercury or higher. Thirteen of the animals were sacrificed. At autopsy, all revealed right ventricular dilatation. In 11 of the entire series, there was slight dilatation; in the remaining 4, the dilata-tion was pronounced. On microscopic examination, the lungs were nor-mal. However, the pulmonary artery and arterioles accompanying the bronchioles were dilated. There was no evidence of hypertrophy of the vessel walls or arteriosclerosis. These animals were studied from 7 to 31 months.[51]

We were so pleased at being able to produce these abnormalities sep-arately that we decided to combine the ventricular septal defect and the pulmonic stenosis. We had five such animals prepared and studied them (for details on one, see Table 14.1). Right-to-left shunting through the defect was demonstrated by the lowering of the percentage of oxygen sat-uration of the systemic (femoral arterial) blood. After eight years of effort, we had very nearly reproduced the tetralogy of Fallot experimentally; a progress report on these and other experiments was sent to Dr. Blalock, who was on vacation, but the studies were never published (see fig. 52).

An interesting and exciting incident occurred during studies on one of the animals in which a high interventricular septal defect had been produced. We were in the process of catheterizing the animal's heart in the fluoroscopic room, which was located on the floor above the operating room. When the catheter was passed into the right side of the heart, it fibrillated. Dr. Kay and I could not have lost more than 10 seconds in

TABLE 14.1:   The Effect on Right Ventricular Pressure and Arterial Oxygen Saturation of the Experimental Production of Pulmonary Stenosis and an Interventricular Septal Defect.

	Pressures in Millimeters of Mercury			
Date	Pulmonary Artery	Right Ventricle[1]	Right Auricle	Arterial O_2 Saturation %
04/30/51	Pulmonary valve cusps and sinuses painted with concentrated nitric acid			
07/24/51[2]	30/10	140/0	20/0	
10/24/51	40/5	120/0	10/0	94.3
10/25/51	Interventricular septal defect produced: ⅛-in. borer			
03/14/52[3]	24/10	110/0	12/0	75.8
05/28/53	15/0	150/0	12/0	
07/27/54	16/0	140/0	14/0	73.4
08/10/54[4]	Dead in a.m.[5]			

[1] The highest right ventricular pressure in 14 dogs in a series in which preoperative pressures were determined was 35 mm. Hg.

[2] Had pronounced systolic murmur from this date.

[3] Marked thrill palpable at fourth interspace.

[4] Animal had remained in remarkably good condition. Had developed no ascites or edema.

[5] Autopsy revealed numerous hemorrhagic areas on surface of lung such as caused by emboli. On opening pulmonary artery at site of stenosis, the area was scarred and had a rough surface with numerous small emboli attached along a band 1 cm. wide in area of the sinuses and remnants of pulmonary valve cusps. The area was fibrous and inelastic. The rim of the interventricular septal defect was smoothly healed and the defect was well placed just below the pulmonary and aortic valve attachments. The right ventricle was markedly hypertrophied.

deciding what to do. I ran downstairs to the operating room to set up a respirator and get a set of surgical instruments. Dr. Kay untied the dog from the fluoroscopic table and brought him down to the operating room, where he was intubated and put on the respirator. The chest was opened immediately and massage of the heart was begun. We estimated a time lapse of three to four minutes from the onset of fibrillation to the beginning of massage. The heart was defibrillated, resulting in a good heart beat in about seven minutes. As the animal was regaining consciousness, he was being slowly anesthetized with ether. The hair was clipped and the area of the incision in the chest was cleaned up as well as possible. After irrigating the chest with antibiotics and saline, leaving some of the antibiotic inside, the chest was closed with interrupted silk sutures. The dog received routine antibiotics for several days and made a complete recovery. The animal was part of the series and subsequent studies were performed. We had made use of the method for defibrillation of the heart that we had so recently developed.

When antibiotics began to be widely used during the mid-1940s, the Professor forbade their use in the laboratory. It was not that he doubted their effectiveness. His concern was that those operating in the laboratory would depend on them instead of adhering to rigid aseptic techniques, a carelessness that might carry over into the general operating rooms.

Our first experience with electronic recording devices was with a Wheatstone bridge, which was designed to be wired into an electro-

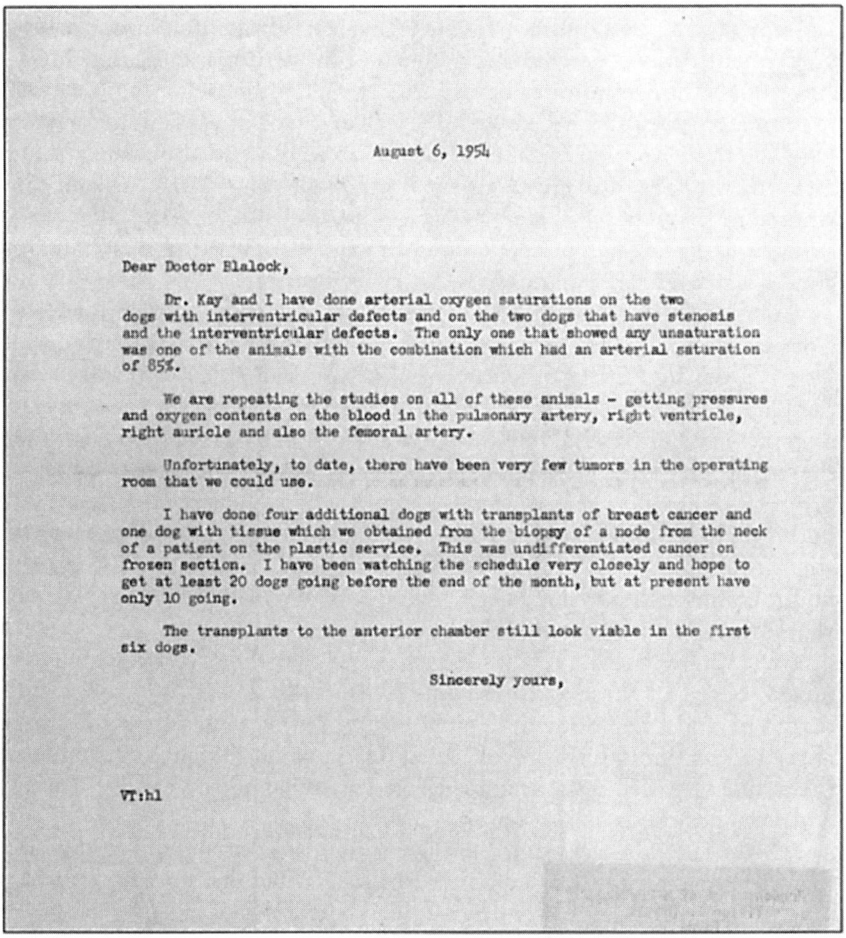

August 6, 1954

Dear Doctor Blalock,

     Dr. Kay and I have done arterial oxygen saturations on the two dogs with interventricular defects and on the two dogs that have stenosis and the interventricular defects. The only one that showed any unsaturation was one of the animals with the combination which had an arterial saturation of 85%.

     We are repeating the studies on all of these animals – getting pressures and oxygen contents on the blood in the pulmonary artery, right ventricle, right auricle and also the femoral artery.

     Unfortunately, to date, there have been very few tumors in the operating room that we could use.

     I have done four additional dogs with transplants of breast cancer and one dog with tissue which we obtained from the biopsy of a node from the neck of a patient on the plastic service. This was undifferentiated cancer on frozen section. I have been watching the schedule very closely and hope to get at least 20 dogs going before the end of the month, but at present have only 10 going.

     The transplants to the anterior chamber still look viable in the first six dogs.

Sincerely yours,

VT:hl

Fig. 52. *Occasionally Dr. Blalock would be out of town for extended periods. This letter to him in 1954 reports his work then in progress while he was away. Numerous other projects are not mentioned in the text or reported in the literature. We were also attempting to transplant carcinomas to the anterior chamber of the eye.*

cardiograph (EKG) machine. To my knowledge, this was the first apparatus for this purpose on the market. We used this method of recording pressures in the numerous cardiac catheterizations we were doing. Each morning, the bridge had to be turned on to warm up for thirty to forty-five minutes, balanced and set for zero on the EKG machine. The pressures were recorded on the EKG paper. Balancing the bridge was often tedious, difficult, and time-consuming.

On one occasion, Dr. Blalock wanted to observe a catheterization so that he could see some of the extremely high right ventricular pressures we were producing with pulmonary stenosis. The Wheatstone bridge lost its adjustment and we were having a difficult time getting it back in balance. After ten or fifteen minutes he whined, "Don't you have a plain mercury manometer and a smoked drum? They always work." Researcher that he was, the Professor was often reluctant to accept new methods and equipment in the laboratory until their worth had been clearly proven. He wanted to know how we were going to record such high ventricular pressures on the narrow EKG paper and we explained how the electronic recorder was calibrated against a mercury manometer.

Other investigations carried out with Dr. Kay were "The Influence of Cortisone and ACTH on the Survival of Adrenal Homotransplants in the Dog"[52] and the "Effect of Sympathectomy on Experimental Frostbite in the Dog."[53] In these latter experiments, I had my first direct contact with a medical student by the name of George D. Zuidema, who was working on the project with us. Neither of us suspected that he would figure so prominently in later years. He was just another medical student, but even in those days my advice to the other technicians was, "If you are going to stay around here, be nice to the students. You don't know which one might come back as your boss." When he returned as my boss thirteen years later, he allowed me to remain.

Dr. Kay wrote the reports for publication as the projects were completed. Seven of these scientific papers were the direct result of the research he and I had done in the laboratory. Dr. Blalock allowed his own name to remain on only one of them and my name to remain on three of them, one of which is the second and last scientific paper that Dr. Blalock and I co-authored.[49]

After Dr. Kay went onto the surgical house staff, he had to take his turn running the cardiac service and being Dr. Blalock's assistant in the "heart room." A few days after doing so, Dr. Kay was to perform a Blalock-Taussig shunt. He took the name of the patient to the Professor, whom he asked to assist him. Dr. Blalock's reply was that he didn't think it would be necessary, since Dr. Kay had spent eighteen months in the laboratory with me. Dr. Blalock never scrubbed with Dr. Kay on any of the numerous operations he performed during his cardiac service. Completing his surgical residency in 1954, Dr. Kay spent two years at the National Heart Institute in Bethesda, Maryland. He was Assistant Clinical Professor of Surgery until 1958 at the University of Southern California School of Medicine in Los Angeles and is now Associate Professor of Surgery.

After completing residency in surgery in 1952, Andrew Glenn Morrow spent a year in thoracic surgery at the General Infirmary in Leeds, England. On returning to the United States and being appointed Chief of Surgery at the National Heart Institute, he was in need of a surgical laboratory technician. He discussed his need with me, saying he did not care to train one, that if he could find someone already trained he could begin his research immediately. He said that he would offer me the job, except his relations with the Professor were good, and that would change if I went with him. He had met Alfred Casper, a chief technician at the old Marine Hospital on Wyman Park Drive. Dr. Morrow had Casper spend time with me to observe and to learn how research and laboratories operate. Casper turned out to be the very person he needed. Dr. Morrow was Chief of Surgery at the National Heart Institute in Bethesda and Associate Professor of Surgery at Johns Hopkins until his death in August 1982, and many of the Hopkins residents had two years of training in cardiac surgery—clinical and research—with him.

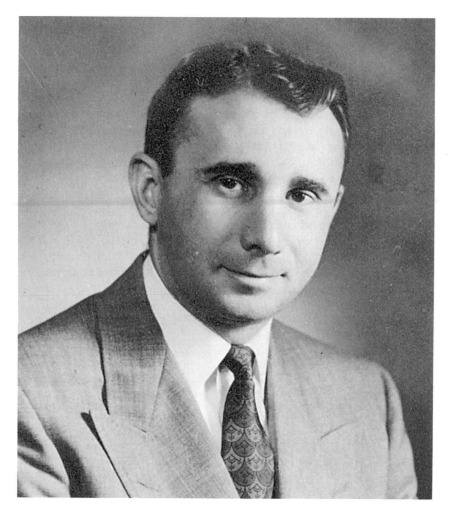

Jerome H. Kay, M.D.

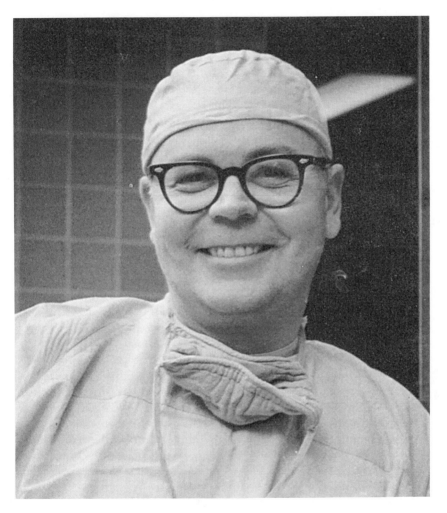

Andrew Glenn Morrow, M.D.

15

Inquiries about the apparatus for positive-pressure anesthesia were still being made in 1948 by visitors to the laboratory. Letters were being sent, some to Dr. Blalock, by doctors who had seen the apparatus, which I had devised, being used in other laboratories. In discussing the demand for the unit with Dr. Johns, the Halsted Fellow in the laboratory, Dr. Hanlon suggested that it might be wise to publish a detailed description so that other institutions with adequate shop facilities could assemble their own. On publication of the description,[29] there was an immediate increase in the number of inquiries instead of the expected decrease. Physicians wanted to know if we could supply the apparatus to them. To accommodate those who had previously requested the unit, I had made good contacts to have the valve machined and motors and other components procured. Allowing myself about one-third the price, I quoted $125 for the first few units I had sent out. When, in 1950, I quoted $145 to Herbert Sloan, M.D., then Professor of Thoracic and Cardiovascular Surgery at the University of Michigan at Ann Arbor, he thought the price was exorbitant until he obtained prices on the components. Earlier, a representative of a company that manufactures medical equipment had asked how much it cost to assemble the unit. When told, he named the price we should have been charging and I was amazed. He explained that the rule was to multiply cost by four or five or even a larger figure if the market would bear it. I assumed from the reaction of Dr. Sloan and others that many of the research laboratories were in the same strained financial condition ours had been and I did not follow the rule. Richard Clay, M.D., who is Clinical Professor of Surgery at the University of Miami, was quoted a price. He wrote back, saying I was a "profiteering burglar," but he bought the anesthesia apparatus. The last unit sent out in 1959 was priced at $210, approximately half the cost of the efficient Harvard respirator, which by then was being widely used. I had supplied over 125 apparatuses for positive-pressure anesthesia to United States laboratories. Three had been sent to Canada and one that required a special motor, to England; a visiting doctor from Brazil took one home with him.

My correspondence was not limited to procurement of the anesthesia apparatus. I became a consultant and general advisor on technical procedure and research projects. Many of the communications covered anything and everything concerning a research laboratory. Doctors who had been residents or had spent a few years on the house staff or as Fellows had questions. These physicians had secured positions, often as heads of departments, at institutions with inadequate research facilities. Some wrote to ask about minor items, but others wanted to know how to start a laboratory. The latter required a list of the equipment and supplies needed for a small laboratory with one or two operating tables, as well as information about sources for large items. Money always seemed to be a problem, and sometimes I was asked to estimate the cost of such a venture. When Arthur Nelson, who is Chief of Surgery at Good Samaritan Hospital in Phoenix, first went to Jacksonville, Florida, he was setting up a laboratory and needed information. When Frank Spencer, who is Professor and Chairman of Surgery at New York University, went to the University of Kentucky as Professor of Surgery our correspondence covered several months. There were many others who consulted me; I considered their requests a compliment and was pleased to give them information.

During the early years, little money was available, and Dr. Blalock was careful about how it was spent. For additional light on the operative field, I had been using a floor-standing goose-neck lamp with a bowl-shaped reflector and 150-watt bulb. When the light was close enough to the field to be of any benefit, the heat it gave off was almost unbearable and the lighting was still inadequate. At Vanderbilt we had used a light worn like the lamp mounted on a coal miner's cap. The strap around the head had to be tight enough to prevent the light from slipping. After an hour or so, one would usually get a terrific headache.

I had struggled through the coarctation project, but while working on the Blue Baby research, I had purchased a portable operating-room light that enabled me to see the fine silk and needles being used. Coming into the laboratory and seeing the light in use, Dr. Blalock asked where I got it. When I told him that he had bought it, he inquired, "I did? How much did I pay for it?"

"Seventy-five dollars," I said. He thought that was a lot of money, but it was actually cheap. The original price quoted was $100. In negotiating and dickering for best prices, for instance, I kept in mind that everything is cheaper by the dozen. Price usually decreases as volume or quantity increases. If I wanted 10 of an item, I would offer half the 20-each price—instead of 10 times the 1-each or 2 times the 5-each. We would receive 10-each of the item and invariably save a few dollars. Sometimes there might be an objection to this way of figuring, but I would chide the company representative, saying they knew only how to add or multiply in pricing but I found it easier to divide. It usually worked.

In purchasing large equipment, it was simplest to have vendors or distributors bid against each other. The large difference between high and low bidder would make one wonder how much a distributor had actually paid for an item. The item from the same manufacturer with the same specifications and the same catalogue number with this wide price range made one question its actual worth.

The big problems in procurement were never with standard supplies and equipment. Research in surgery and physiology happens to be a field of "gadgetry." Doctors and investigators like to visit other laboratories and hospitals, where they collect sample gadgets and/or instruments they would like to use in their studies. A doctor would give me his sample and tell me he wanted a new one, or perhaps six or two dozen. If it was large enough, it might have identifying marks such as a manufacturer's name or a number. If it was small, more than likely it had been removed from its original packaging and had no identifying marks. Then I would have to find out what it was, what it was used for, who made it, and who sold it. If the doctor didn't know, the catalogue search began. To order it, I needed the catalogue number. If it was a new item, it might not be in a catalogue. Then I would take it to central supply, the source of a great variety of hospital and laboratory supplies. If they couldn't identify it, I would call a company representative who might be able to do so. He would arrive and say, "Oh, that's a so-and-so." Then he would give me the price, ask how many I wanted, and tell me when he could make delivery. At this point, I didn't even dicker about price.

An amusing, but rather difficult, request was made by Mr. Phillip Allison from Oxford, England, who was Visiting Professor of Surgery. He worked in the department for two or three months. He asked if I would get him some "soft paraffin" and I told him I'd be happy to. I looked in the catalogue of histological supplies. I had construed soft paraffin to mean soft at room temperature. The catalogue listed no paraffin that melted below 275°F. I went back to Mr. Allison several days later and asked what the melting point of the paraffin he'd requested was, that I could not locate any with a very low melting point. He smilingly told me, "Oh, it's common, you can get it at the drugstore," asking himself, "Oh, what do you call it?" then, thinking intensely to himself, he says, "Vaseline." Imagine my embarrassment, or was it he who should have been embarrassed?

Sometimes an investigator would get information about an item he wanted, and the information was often incomplete. If the item had been custom made, it was simply a matter of contacting the proper shop in the Hopkins medical complex to have it duplicated. There were all kinds of shops, mechanical and electronic with highly skilled technicians who could duplicate just about anything or make solid realities of any ideas the numerous investigators might have. I was expected to know about thousands of items used in the laboratory. With the rapidly changing times and technology and the increase in volume and scope of research in the field, it was difficult to keep pace.

It took many years for salesmen and vendor representatives to adjust to the fact that I was the responsible person with whom they would have to do business for the laboratory. I could be talking with a student, doctor, or one of the laboratory personnel and salesmen would approach and, looking at him, ask if he was Mr. Thomas. It never occurred to them that the name Mr. Thomas indicated no particular color. With me sitting at the desk in the office and no one else present, it was not unusual for a salesman to look in the door and ask if Mr. Thomas was in or if I knew where he was. My usual response was, "Sure, he's sitting right here." It was amusing to watch their reaction, many becoming very red faced.

Shortly after Dr. Hanlon had become the official director of the laboratory, a salesman came into the laboratory. Seeing him in the hallway, I asked if I could help him. He said, "Sure you can help me. You can tell me where I can find the doctor who's in charge of the laboratory." I gave him the name of the doctor, the building, and the room number in the hospital where his office was located. I knew that if he had any intention of supplying anything to the laboratory, the chances were 99 to 1 that he'd be back to talk with me. I also knew that in the manner he'd responded to my question, he'd just talked himself into an embarrassing situation. About 45 minutes later, he returned. This time he wanted to know where he would find Mr. Thomas. I told him that he'd just found him. It was obvious from the way he blushed that he'd been given a name but not a race. Hesitantly and sheepishly, he asked why I hadn't told him that I did the purchasing for the laboratory. I smilingly told him the answer was very simple; he had asked a specific question and I had given a specific answer. Despite incidents such as these, salesmen and I developed a good rapport and many friendships were formed. I couldn't hold the company representatives accountable for their reactions to such a drastic change in Hopkins personnel.

During the early years at Hopkins, some of the Professor's visits to the laboratory would be as short as five or ten minutes. By the early to mid-1950s, he seemed to be getting some of the pressure off his time. Instead of coming in for a few minutes to get experimental results or have a short discussion, he began to participate actively in the research. This seemed to have been one of his most relaxed periods during his entire administration. The stress of operating daily on high-risk cardiac patients had taken its toll on him. His youthful appearance on arrival at Hopkins in 1941, when he had been mistaken for one of the house officers by a nurse on Halsted, had now given way to the more professorial look. Now he was more at ease and seemed to thoroughly enjoy himself. He was doing what was his second nature, or possibly his first nature, research.

Sometimes he would come into the laboratory and sit at the desk for as long as half an hour studying notes and protocols, while I was busy in the operating room at the opposite end of the building. He would write notes and comment on his impression gleaned from my protocols. In the laboratory he had time to concentrate on his research without being disturbed.

In conversations that might follow, he was usually relaxed and pleasant, but still the pure scientist—the subject being the active projects, some possible new approach to them, or an approach to a new project. These were the conversations in which he might say, "I wonder what would happen if you did so and so?" or "Sometime when you get a chance, why don't you try so and so?" He seldom went into much detail as to how anything was to be done. I would have to make notes of such statements because, however minor they might seem, he would remember them. If I hadn't mentioned the results of the trials, months later he would ask as if he'd suddenly remembered, "Oh! What happened when you tried so and so?" He used this method of issuing instructions throughout the department and found it very effective, his "I wonder" being translated to mean, "I want you to find out," and "when you get a chance," to "Take the time to try it."

At times, Dr. Blalock would come into the laboratory and assist in whatever procedure was in progress. As time passed, he began to have specific procedures scheduled for himself. Occasionally, he'd be on a rigid schedule and would state beforehand that his time was limited. This meant having the given procedure at a certain stage when he arrived, which called for accurate timing on our part. A good percentage of the procedures he scheduled for himself were not part of any ongoing research project. He was usually noncommittal when scheduling, thus leaving me at a loss as to whether some of the procedures were practice sessions for surgery he planned to perform on patients, whether he was determining feasibility, or whether he was merely trying out his skills. Having no direct contact with the operating room in the hospital at the time, I had no way of knowing if he used any of these procedures clinically.

He had me prepare a series of animals with interventricular septal defects so that he could attempt closures. In one method of closure, he would blindly wedge a cone-shaped plug of polyvinyl sponge in the defect. This was accomplished by first placing a purse-string suture isolating an area in the left auricular wall. A heavy guide suture on a large curved liver needle was passed into the left auricle through the isolated auricular wall and through the mitral orifice, into the left ventricle, through the septal defect, and out through the wall of the right ventricle. The smaller end of the cone-shaped prosthesis was tied onto the trailing heavy suture. An incision was made in the left auricle within the purse-string suture and the prosthesis pulled into the auricle by traction on the needle end of the suture. The purse-string suture was tied. The plug of polyvinyl sponge was then pulled through the mitral orifice and into the septal defect until the harsh thrill on the right side of the heart was obliterated. The compressibility of the sponge had been underestimated in the first experiments and the plug was forced through the defect. With much larger plugs the method was successful in only two instances. Both animals died within a few days due to partial blockage of the aortic orifice. There was no way to anchor a smaller sponge in place. The heart-lung machine was still in the development stage. Later, in several animals, he placed the mitral valve prosthesis (polyvinyl sponge), the technique that Dr. Johns had developed. Dr. Blalock also performed closures of interatrial septal defects by several methods, including the Crafoord technique.

The Professor would at times have general discussions with the other investigators or their Fellows about their projects, their procedures, their results, and the problems encountered, and he would offer suggestions. He was well informed and kept abreast of the findings in most of the research projects being carried out in the laboratory. At times, he would talk with the other technicians or laboratory assistants about projects on which they were working. The fact that Dr. Blalock talked with them and asked questions had a positive effect, thus they took a more active interest in their research projects.

I had never thought of myself as or cared to be a supervisor of personnel, and Dr. Blalock's personal contact with the laboratory personnel certainly made the task easier. With the responsibility thrust upon me, I had to develop a philosophy and work out a system for dealing with the people under my supervision. I didn't have the time for and could not afford personnel problems. I had always worked with a minimum of supervision and had a thorough dislike for supervisors and supervision. I disliked giving orders and telling people what to do. I felt then, as I do now, that more can be gained by teaching people to do what is required and expected, and then putting the responsibility for performance on them. Furthermore, no one worked for me. They all worked for the Johns Hopkins University, in the Department of Surgery, under the Professor. I just happened to be the person the Professor had put in charge of the laboratory and I was responsible to him. In the laboratory they would be working with me. The *with* was very important, inasmuch as there was no opposite position to take, whereas if they were supposed to be work-ing *for* me, they might take the opposite position and work against me.

On only a few occasions did I have to explain my philosophy to em-ployees, letting them know my responsibility, what was expected of them, and what would and would not be tolerated. Very few problems arose. They accepted their responsibility, and the vast majority liked it that way and worked *with* me.

The technical help in the laboratory received on-the-job training. When additional or replacement help was required, I would move my as-sistant into the vacancy and train the new employee myself. In many in-stances, it was impossible to keep some of the better and more promising men in the laboratory because of the ridiculously low pay scale. This was particularly true immediately following World War II. With the return of the surgical staff and the increase in the amount of research, I was hard pressed to keep pace with the need for additional laboratory personnel. I talked with Dr. Blalock on several occasions to get him to raise the sala-ries of individuals who would be assets to the laboratory, but I was never successful. Neither he nor the institution seemed to realize that you get the quality of personnel you are willing to pay for.

Essentially, these laboratory assistants were put through the same type of training I had received at Vanderbilt in the early 1930s. I was with them most of each day, thereby making their training intensive. During the early period, I would teach them what would be required, letting them know that if they didn't like the job they were free to leave. A few left because they couldn't cope with the odors or the sight of blood. If, on the other hand, they failed to show sufficient interest or cooperation, they were told of their shortcomings and let go.

Once a laboratory assistant was trained, there was little excuse for his not carrying out his assignments. I was almost always available and the technical staff was always very cooperative in helping one another. They had been taught to administer anesthesia, inhalation or intravenous, how to prepare operative fields for aseptic procedures, and how to set up and sterilize surgical instruments. They were also taught how to set up for acute experiments and how to care for apparatus and equipment after its use. If there was no Fellow or student working with me, the laboratory assistant would be taught to scrub up and assist on experimental surgical procedures. Later they would be allowed to make the incision with my assistance. When they eventually made the incision alone, I performed the procedure, and they closed the incisions, which enabled me to write operative notes and take care of administrative duties.

I never hesitated to promote the laboratory assistants or surgical technicians. When asked about procurng a technician to work in or head a laboratory elsewhere, I first inquired as to the salary offered. If it was higher than that being paid by Hopkins, I would recommend someone from our technical staff.

One such incident happened with Julius Mayo. In 1956 Dr. Mark M. Ravitch became Chief of Surgery at Baltimore City Hospitals, which lacked facilities and personnel for surgical research. Dr. Ravitch immediately proceeded to set up a laboratory and secure needed personnel. When Dr. Ravitch asked for help for his laboratory, Julius Mayo was sent to Baltimore City Hospitals.

Mayo had been an orderly in the general operating rooms during the integration of operating-room personnel at Hopkins. The locker rooms and rest rooms for the orderlies were located on the same floor as the operating rooms, but the colored men coming into the system were required to use locker rooms on the basement level. Mayo let it be known that he did not agree with the arrangement. Being the only one to voice his displeasure, he was considered a potential troublemaker and pressured to leave. Not being intimidated, he was eventually fired, after which I took him into the laboratory and trained him. Dr. Blalock soon missed Mayo and asked why I had let him go. I told him that a better salary had been offered. Dr. Blalock and I had discussed laboratory salaries so many times that he made no comment.

After the stint at Baltimore City Hospitals, Mayo eventually came back to our laboratory, but has since returned to Baltimore City Hospitals in the neurosurgical laboratory with Dr. Gunduz Gucer, who completed his neurosurgical residency at Hopkins in 1976.

Numerous surgical technicians who received their training in the Surgical Research Laboratory at Hopkins were placed in other departments and institutions. Freddie Jackson, who went to Baltimore City Hospitals with Dr. William Milnor, is back at Hopkins, still with Milnor in the department of physiology. William Cooper went to the biomedical engineering laboratory at Hopkins with Dr. Donald Gann, but has since left the field. William Petty is with Dr. Clarence Weldon, who is now Chief of the Division of Cardiothoracic Surgery at Washington University in Saint Louis.

Raymond Lee began working for Hopkins as an elevator operator in Halsted. After talking with him on several occasions while riding the elevator, I asked if he might not be interested in becoming a laboratory assistant. When a vacancy occurred, I brought him into the laboratory in 1963. After he worked there for several years, he was asked to join Dr. Henry Bahnson, who is Professor and Chairman of Surgery at the University of Pittsburgh. Raymond spent a year at Pittsburgh before returning to Hopkins. As physician's assistant, he is an integral part of the clinical cardiovascular surgical team under Dr. Vincent Gott, Chief of Cardio-vascular Division of Surgery. Another of the "graduate technicians" from the Surgical Research Laboratory at Hopkins in 1972 was Jake McLaughlin, who worked with Dr. David Skinner. When Skinner left Hopkins to become Professor of Surgery at the University of Chicago, Jake went to the Hopkins clinical transplantation surgical service. As a physician's assistant, he holds a responsible position on the kidney transplant team under Dr. G. Melville Williams, Professor of Transplantation Surgery.

Throughout the years, I tried to have a summer position available for a high-school student who was interested in research or medicine. Two such students, James Ralph and John Johnson, went on to earn their doctorates in medicine.

Two extremely good technicians, John Gary and William Gardner, left because of their salaries, the level of which I had discussed with Dr. Blalock. Both had taken unbelievable initiative in their work. Always a step ahead of their co-workers, anticipating every possible move and need, they went on to more financially promising fields.

Most laboratory personnel were hired in their late teens or early twenties, with at least a high-school education. If a problem could not be resolved, they would be told to find another job. I would explain that it was too early in their careers to have "fired" on an employment record. On one occasion, I was having difficulty with a technician that Dr. Blalock liked. When I told Dr. Blalock that I would have to let him go, his response was, "Do whatever you want to. It's easy to hire and fire, but getting work out of people is a little difficult. You spend a lot of time training these people." I told the technician about the conversation with Dr. Blalock. He thought it over and I did not have to ask him to find another job. The records of those who worked with me in the laboratory show that only one was fired, and that was for dishonesty. Other reasons for termination were "quit to take another job," "going back to school" (which I encouraged), or "personal reasons."

By the mid- to late-1960s the institution had adjusted salaries to a more satisfactory level. However, we were still dealing with people. One very independent technician who knew he was good began setting a bad pattern of conduct and work habits. I had numerous conversations with him, but there was no change in his conduct or attitude. When, as a last resort, I told him he would have to find another job, he laughed and walked out of the office. He went to the doctor to whose research team he had been assigned and told his part of the story. At the request of the investigator, I was in a conference with him within twenty-four hours. I explained that there were seven other technicians on the floor at the time. If he could get away with poor conduct, why couldn't the others? The technician was given two months in which to assist in the completion of a research project. After hearing he had two months, he sheepishly told me he hadn't thought I could fire him. I could only ask how he had reasoned that I had the authority to hire him but not to fire him.

There was very little discussion of administrative matters between Dr. Blalock and me although I usually kept him informed of matters I felt were important. On occasions, matters would arise that I thought were above and beyond my duty, responsibility, or authority. When I presented such matters to Dr. Blalock, he almost invariably replied, "That's your job. Do whatever you think or settle it any way you want to. I have enough problems of my own." Receiving this type of reply on numerous occasions, I began making my own decisions in many matters in which I thought my authority and/or judgment might be questioned. I would inform him later, but he never questioned my decisions.

16

The laboratory was a separate structure in the Hopkins medical complex; access from the hospital was overland and across two streets. There was also a service tunnel, by way of the power and heating plant, that I used during the winter on extremely inclement days. Between the Medical School and the power plant, there was a change in the level of the tunnel at which a six- to eight-foot ladder had to be negotiated. This feature may have discouraged its use because I seldom encountered anyone in the tunnel.

During World War II, on a cold, wintry day with several inches of snow on the ground, Dr. Blalock made one of his visits to the laboratory. He came down the hallway stomping his feet and shaking his coat to dislodge the snow. Getting just inside the laboratory door, he looked at his watch and asked, "Why the hell did I come over here. I'm due somewhere else. I'll see you next time." He turned and left. Tom and I looked at each other and laughed, with Tom jokingly commenting, "That man sure doesn't trust you. No reason he would possibly come out in this gosh awful weather except to check up on you." ("Gosh awful" was about the extent of Tom's profanity.)

I relate this incident to emphasize Dr. Blalock's devotion to the laboratory and research. Come hell or high water (snow or sleet, in this instance), he would find his way to the laboratory.

With the importance he attached to research, Dr. Blalock was unhappy about the distance that had to be traversed and the amount of time consumed to get to and from the Hunterian building, "the dog house." The situation was not conducive to the use of the laboratory by the doctors in clinical practice, or by those in training in the hospital. The trip from office to laboratory and return required fifteen to twenty minutes, depending upon elevator service and the location of one's office in the hospital. His feeling, often expressed, was that with sufficient technical help in the laboratory to prepare for the arrival of anyone who wanted to work, this wasted time could be used in productive research if the laboratory were more easily accessible.

A heroic plan for the rebuilding of the hospital was undertaken in 1950. The first building in the plan, called Reconstruction Unit #1 (RU-1), was to replace the old surgical building that still housed radiology and the accident room. When wrecking of the building began, I expressed the opinion that I would probably be walking with a cane by the time the new building was erected. Even though by this time much was being done to improve the facilities, my original impression of Johns Hopkins had not been dispelled; thus I was surprised when trucks began bringing concrete and pouring footings for the new structure even before debris of the old building was cleared away. Dr. Blalock had played an important role in the project, and the problem of the accessibility of the animal research laboratory was to be resolved. Along with his other efforts, he designated $150,000 from the by then well-filled coffers of the department of surgery to be used in the financing of the construction of RU-1. These funds had accrued from the professional fees of the department, mostly for heart operations. The building, a thirteen-story structure, was to house animal research facilities on the eleventh, twelfth, and thirteenth floors. The entire building was "shelled in," but originally only the first, second, fifth, and sixth floors were completed and occupied.

The department of surgery was ultimately to occupy the twelfth and thirteenth floors for development of the surgical research laboratories. Planning for the research facilities was well under way in fall 1953. The architects and hospital planners had been working with Dr. Blalock, Dr. Bahnson, and myself in the department. By this time, Dr. Ravitch, who had worked on the overall planning of the new building, had gone to Mount Sinai Hospital in New York as Director of Surgery. Dr. Ravitch had been appointed to work with the architects to design an emergency room, offices, and laboratories, seeing to it that the requirements of the surgical staff, investigators, and the department of anesthesia were met. This assignment included providing details of how each room was to be equipped and used. He also contributed to the general layout of the twelfth (laboratory) floor. Drs. Blalock and Ravitch had keenly felt the need for an additional large classroom, such as Hurd Hall, which they thought should be in a surgical area. This, of course, would occupy substantial space at the expense of the department. A quadrangle is formed by Osler, Halsted, the dispensary building, and the corridor. The area had no real access; windows on basement levels were in wells and those on the first floor were not in use. Almost leisurely observing from a window overlooking this scene, Dr. Ravitch realized that this was the place for the new classroom. When he went to the Professor and made the suggestion, Dr. Blalock liked the idea and immediately went into action. With the Professor's influence, the new auditorium, sometimes referred to as the poor man's Hurd Hall, was incorporated in the building project within days.

Dr. Blalock had an opportunity to tour the research building at the Mayo Clinic in mid-November 1953 and was impressed by their animal cages and care facilities. On his return, he had all architectural and engineering work suspended on the thirteenth floor for a complete reevaluation of the animal-care and other laboratory areas. He stated that as long as we were going to spend almost $2 million in developing the facilities, there was no excuse not to do it right and get the very best for the money. He couldn't wait to send a team to Mayo to study the design, construction, and operation of their animal-care and research facilities. The team included Thomas Silcox, an architect from James R. Edmunds Associates; Henry J. Gaffney, an engineer; and me. Until then I had spent only limited time on the project. Dr. Blalock didn't care to see his research slow down, but with this development I became involved to the extent that research was halted for about three months.

The trip would have been a week earlier, but Thanksgiving intervened. Arriving in Rochester on December 2, Dr. John H. Grindley, the Director of Surgical Research of the Mayo Clinic, was our host. Besides being available himself, he had made arrangements for us to consult with their engineers. Many others who were involved in the operation of the laboratory were also available to answer questions. Silcox and Gaffney, architect and engineer, were to study the design and construction of the animal-care area; then we were to observe the operation of the facilities and judge the practicality of the installation. The assignment was enormous in this specially designed area, for the caging of dogs involved special floor construction for drainage. In this area we observed their methods of cleaning, food preparation, and the actual feeding and watering of the animals. We also inspected the facilities for the caging of small animals. Along with visiting these animal-care areas, I had been instructed to observe and ask about the use of the research areas. This included the layout of the laboratories; equipment, operating tables, lighting, and methods of handling and preparing animals for surgery; the types and methods of administering anesthesia; the preparation of sterile supplies; and the overall operation of the research laboratories.

It had been a whirlwind tour, but through the courtesy and cooperation of Dr. Grindley we had a fruitful visit to the research building. In less than two days, we had amassed an enormous amount of information that was most valuable to us in the development of our facilities. We returned by way of Chicago, stopping long enough to tour the animal facilities at the University of Chicago. We found that their animal-care area had been developed along the same lines as those we had seen at the Mayo Clinic.

The new surgical research laboratories were ready for occupancy the last week of March 1955. With only three class sessions remaining in that quarter of the school year, we decided to postpone the move until they were completed. We estimated that it would require three days to move equipment, supplies, and animals. This was scheduled for April 20, 21, and 22, and we were to use the hospital truck and the laboratory technical personnel. The truck and its driver, Larrette ("Slim") Whittaker, were available from 7 a.m. to 4 p.m. The laboratory technical staff hours were from 9 a.m. to 5 p.m. I was concerned that we'd have a six-hour work day if everyone insisted on getting a one-hour lunch break. The laboratory staff, however, agreed to come in at 7 a.m. On the first day at about 3 p.m., when I thought they'd all be ready to quit for the day, they decided to complete the move of supplies and equipment. It was completed shortly after 7 p.m.

At 7 a.m. the following morning, everyone was ready to move the animals. There were 120 dogs to be moved into the new quarters and individual cages. The identifying and marking systems were completely different in the old and new areas. Each animal had to be identified by number, investigator's name, room number, and cage number, keeping each investigator's animals in the same room. I'd had several sessions with the laboratory personnel about problems that might be encountered and had given them the responsibility of working out a method. They split themselves into two teams of three each, with Claude Brown heading the shipping group in the old laboratory and William Gardner heading the team on the receiving end in the new quarters. At about 6 p.m. spot checks of the animals in the new cages revealed no errors in identification. I thanked them for a job well done and told them I'd see them Monday. Someone said "Tomorrow is Friday." I said I knew that and would see them Monday. There was a chorus of "Oh, thank you."

On Friday morning, I went in early. Every large piece of equipment had been tagged, and every box containing instruments and supplies had been marked with a room number. Everything had been placed in its assigned room. By midmorning I had unpacked the office and was ready for business. I was in the central support area unpacking instruments and supplies when Dr. Blalock arrived. He immediately noticed that no one was around. I told him that because they'd worked conscientiously for two twelve-hour days instead of the three days we'd estimated, I had given them the day off. Unhappily, he whined, "Well, just because they worked a few hours overtime was no reason to give them a day off." I said I knew that, but I was the one who had to work with them every day. He asked when I expected to get work started, and I told him two operations were scheduled for Monday morning. This, of course, pleased him immmensely.

Johns Hopkins is a teaching and research institution, but the far greater proportion of the activity in the laboratory is research. Medical-School students learned operative surgery in the old Hunterian Laboratory (see fig. 53). The large operating-room area that formed the core of the new facilities was more spacious and attractive than that in the old laboratory. The walls were light green ceramic tile; the ceiling was sus-

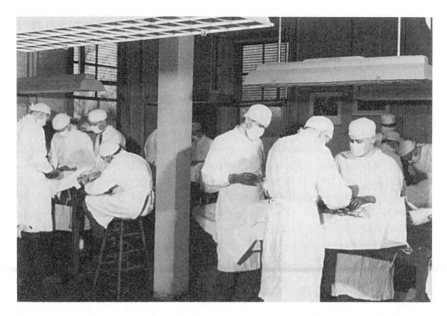

Fig. 53. Students at work in the last class in operative (dog) surgery held in the old Hunterian Laboratory. Dr. Joseph Miller, one of the instructors, is seen third from left standing behind second student. I am in the background at right. The fluorescent lights had been installed only a few years earlier. Courtesy J. Lindsay Burch.

pended fibre tile and the floor, a pre-waxed vinyl tile. The size of the laboratory allowed for more ease of movement between the operating tables, which were custom made. The stainless-steel tops were V-shaped with an inch-wide slot at the bottom of the V for drainage and ease of cleaning. A removable trough, to catch waste, ran beneath this slot for the length of the table. The legs, with adjustable leveling feet, were of two-inch galvanized pipe that was painted aluminum. With a few modifications the design was very similar to that of the wooden tables in the old laboratory. Three of the eight tables had ceiling-mounted lights. Portable lights on floor stands were provided at the remaining tables, and there were standard surgical instrument tables with stainless steel tops.

The services, electricity, suction, and compressed air were supplied from the ceiling on a pendant near the head of each table. Electricity was supplied at the foot of each table in a similar manner. The area was also used for research, which, in the old laboratory, could not be scheduled on afternoons when class sessions were held. It was desirable to correct that situation, so a secondary operating room with three tables was included.

One support or work room served both operating rooms. Autoclaves and sterilizers were kept there, and the area was used for the preparation and sterilization of the operating-room supplies and instruments. We no longer had to use the fish-kettle boilers to sterilize the surgical instruments, since they could be sterilized in autoclaves at a temperature of 240°F. Most of the chronic aseptic procedures were confined to these central-core operating rooms.

This large classroom area also had another important function. New surgical procedures and techniques developed in this and similar surgical research and experimental surgery laboratories are reported in medical journals, along with the results of the clinical use of such procedures. Detailed descriptions with illustrations are usually presented so that surgeons will have access to the new procedures and techniques for use in the treatment of their own patients. Surgeons frequently would come to the laboratory, with journal in hand, to become familiar with a procedure before attempting it on a patient.

A corridor bordered this central classroom area, and on the periphery were individual laboratories and office spaces. There were separate laboratories for chemistry, physiology, bacteriology, and histology, as well as an X-ray and fluoroscopy room with a darkroom for processing film. An incinerator for the disposal of dead animals and waste material from the laboratory was located on the fourteenth-floor level off the elevator tower and the mechanical services area.* Animals were delivered on the basement level at an entrance near the base of the freight elevator shaft and carried up, express, to the thirteenth-floor animal-care area.

Within days of moving and performing a few aseptic surgical procedures, we found that the iodine and alcohol being used to prepare the skin of our animals for surgery was damaging the tops of our stainless-steel operating tables. Our "prep" solution was immediately changed to a solution that contained acetone and alcohol, both of which are highly volatile and flammable. About a week later someone had been too liberal in pouring the solution in preparation for an operative procedure, and the excess solution had run into the trough and then the waste bucket beneath the table. The Professor visited the laboratory during the procedure and, standing near the foot of the table, lit a cigarette. He casually flicked his match into the waste bucket, setting off a huge flash of flame. The bucket was removed and the fire was extinguished before any damage was done. Dr. Blalock, who was badly shaken, ordered me to post No Smoking signs and read them to anyone caught smoking in the area. I was to report anyone who refused to obey the signs.

*Use of the incinerator has since been discontinued to meet clean-air standards.

Mr. Alan V. Pollock, Traveling Fellow in Surgery from the United Leeds Hospital in England, arrived to work with us in July 1954. He was a proper English gentleman, rather quiet but pleasant, a very personable chap with a wry sense of humor. The English call their doctors *Mister*, and he told me that if your professor called you *Doctor*, he did not hold you in very high esteem at the moment.

One of his major research projects was a continuing effort to find a suitable method for the surgical treatment of valvular heart disease. In these experiments, transplants of homologous cusps of the tricuspid valve were performed.[54] Much of the experimental work on valve replacement had been done on the tricuspid valve because of the ease of access. Also, such a procedure could be carried out in this area of the heart without the danger of systemic air embolism before the perfection of the heart-lung machine (extracorporeal circulation).

To obtain the valve cusps, a dog under Nembutal anesthesia was heparinized and bled into bottles. The blood was used for perfusion of the recipient during implantation of the cusps. The antero-superior cusp of the tricuspid valve was removed aseptically and kept in a pan of sterile saline until ready for use about thirty minutes later.

Under aseptic conditions the right or left carotid artery of the recipient was cannulated in the central direction. Under positive-pressure ether anesthesia, the heart was exposed and appropriate ligatures and umbilical tapes were placed around the major vessels to temporarily occlude the circulation and isolate the heart. Perfusion with the heparinized arterial blood was begun through the carotid cannula at a rate of about fifty millimeters per minute. Tapes on the cavae were tightened to occlude the inflow of blood to the heart. The aortic tape was used to exclude the lower part of the body from the perfusion. The right atrium was incised and the antero-superior cusp of the tricuspid valve was removed under direct vision. The homograft cusp was inserted into the right ventricle, and its papillary muscle was fastened to the papillary muscle of the recipient with a silk suture. A continuous silk suture was used to unite the fibrous base of the graft to the fibrous annulus at the site of the removed cusp. The right side of the heart was allowed to fill with blood, a Pott's clamp was applied to temporarily close the incision in the right atrium and all the tapes removed. The time of cardiac occlusion was eight to ten minutes. The atrium was closed with a continuous silk suture. The results were not encouraging. In only four out of ten experiments was the competence of the valve moderate to good. All the transplanted cusps showed opacity, thickening, and loss of resilience.

To those of us who had endured life in the old building, moving to this new laboratory was a blessing. The old dog house had whatever temperature prevailed outside—the windows were so loose fitting that they rattled when the wind blew. During cold winter weather, we worked with sweaters or jackets beneath scrub suits and gowns. On several occasions, I had closed the laboratory because of the bitter cold and sent everyone home. In summer the temperature was at the other extreme. Added to the heat from outside was the heat from an autoclave and from fish-kettle boilers for sterilizing surgical instruments. On three occasions the fire sprinkler system went off. The first was an unforgettable experience. I was operating, wearing no undershirt, but had ʼned cap, mask, gown, and gloves. For additional light, I was using a goose-neck lamp. I was extremely warm, so I had Tom move the light. He was giving anesthesia and occasionally mopping perspiration from my brow, which might otherwise have dripped onto the operative field. There was a pop like the sound of a .22-caliber rifle being fired directly over our heads. Tom ran for the doorway. About the time I looked around to see where he was going in such a hurry, I had what seemed like a barrel of water dumped on me from above. Running to the hallway where Tom stood, I asked why he didn't tell me to run. When he controlled his laughter, he said he didn't have time but that next time I heard the shot, I'd know I was supposed to run. The Medical-School engineers had heard an alarm outside the building. The weather being so hot, they knew what it was and cut off the sprinkler system in a few minutes.

The course in operative surgery, usually referred to as "dog surgery," is the first training in surgery that medical students receive and is offered as an elective in their junior year. Over 95 percent of the students in each class sign up for this course, in which they actually perform surgical procedures. Each class is instructed by at least two part-time surgical staff members.

Each class is divided into teams of four: the surgeon, his first assistant, the instrument nurse, and the anesthetist. Positions on the team are rotated each session, thus allowing every student to perform in each capacity. During the 1940s, sessions were held twice weekly. Four dogs were assigned to each team, and two weeks would elapse between operative procedures on any one dog. Later, when sessions were reduced to once a week, only two dogs were assigned to a team. These dogs were the patients of the team, which was held accountable for their survival and health. Preoperative medication was given to the animals by one of the technical staff. Ether was the anesthetic agent, administered by the open-drop method until early in the 1970s, being the only agent with which the stages of anesthesia could be demonstrated. Considering the danger of explosion and the fire hazard inherent in the use of ether, it was decided to change to an intravenous agent.

While we were still occupying the old building, a representative of the Mine Safety Corporation came into the laboratory to promote a company product, the Neophore, for use in positive-pressure anesthesia. Class was in session and the students were administering ether by the open-drop method. His first question was whether we'd ever had a fire or an explosion. His judgment was that there was enough ether vapor in the building to blow it up with all of us in it. Fortunately, we never had a fire or explosion, probably because we were careful. Our supply of ether and acetone was stored in a wooden shed in a walled courtyard outside the building.

The students were taught general operating-room dress, the wearing of caps and masks, aseptic technique, how to scrub for surgery, how to don gown and gloves, how to prepare the patient's skin, and how to drape the operative site. They learned to restrict their movements to avoid contaminating themselves and the operative field. They were taught how to tie knots and how to use surgical instruments, and as Halsted had emphasized, the gentle handling of tissue.

A demonstration of each operative procedure was performed by the instructors, who explained each step in minute detail. At the next session, the students would repeat the procedure with the instructors looking over their shoulders, verbally coaching them. With six to eight teams operating simultaneously, it was almost impossible for the two assigned instructors to cover all of them on some of the procedures. With some of the pairs of instructors, it was not unusual for only one to be present, and sometimes I would be left alone with the students. Even though I seldom participated in the demonstrations, I was always looking over a shoulder, helping to coach them. Only on rare occasions was it necessary to don gloves to get them out of difficulty, this usually being profuse bleeding that the student couldn't control.

The first session for each group was always indoctrination. The laboratory accommodated a maximum of eight separate teams simultaneously. The overall responsibility for the class was mine, but despite all the organization, planning, and preparation, there would still be a good deal of confusion during the second session. The students would come in, get as many as eight dogs, to restrain on operating tables, and anesthetize them. At the same time, the other twenty or more students would come in ready to don caps and masks and scrub up. Most of the students would have to be re-instructed in what to do and how to do it. To get the teams ready to begin the operations would usually require all the technical help available. Tom used to say that a record should have played continuously, giving instructions as to what each student should do.

With dog-surgery classes being held twice weekly, the schedule of operations to be performed by the students was extensive. The schedule included the following procedures: nerve suture, tendon suture (Achilles tendon), thyroidectomy, splenectomy, nephrectomy, cholecystectomy, pneumonectomy, intestinal resection, and a caecectomy (appendectomy). During the last session of each class, amputations were performed, after which the animals were sacrificed and autopsies performed. Operative and follow-up notes were required on each animal. At autopsy, the sites of the various procedures were examined and the findings written up in a report. If an animal died during the course, autopsies were required to determine the cause of death.

Dr. Ferdinand Lee, the primary instructor for many years, was strict, demanding, and very effective. He taught not only surgical techniques, but also postoperative care and physical signs. He would make the rounds of each team, usually while the incision was being closed, and inquire about the condition of the other patients: their physical appearance; whether they were eating, drinking, vomiting (after intestinal resection), able to walk (after tendon suture); and how their wounds were healing.

On Dr. Lee's retirement in 1946, Dr. Edward Stafford was put in charge of the course. Among those working with him at various times over a period of many years were Drs. George Finney, Sr.; William F. Rienhoff, Jr.; I. Ridgeway Trimble; Joseph Miller; William F. Rienhoff III; Jacob C. Handelsman; William E. Grose; John Classen; Alan C. Woods, Jr.; and others. Dr. Woods was put in charge of the course in 1963. Joining him with some of the preceding were Drs. Theodore Wilson, Marvin Nachlas, and Paul Leand.

With the change from the semester system to the trimester and later back to the quarter system, the schedule of operations to be performed by the medical students had to be drastically reduced in number and variety. About the time of the change to the quarter system and the advent of cardiac and vascular surgery, a blood-vessel anastomosis was added to the schedule.

17

Henry T. Bahnson, after graduating from Harvard in 1944, had begun his surgical training as an intern at Hopkins. Denton Cooley was also an intern. It was difficult for interns and members of the house staff to find time to work in the laboratory, but these two succeeded. Working at night, they performed a series of experiments on wringer (washing-machine) injuries. Alternating in watching their animals throughout the night, they rarely got much sleep. Dr. Bahnson also found time a few years later to practice vascular suturing by performing subclavian-to-pumonary-artery anastomoses, as had been done at Vanderbilt in earlier attempts to produce pulmonary hypertension. His interest in cardio-vascular surgery was so great that he began working in the laboratory almost immediately upon completion of his residency in 1951. Many investigators were working on the development and perfection of a pump oxygenator for use in open-heart surgery. Dr. Bahnson began by trying rotating disks as an oxygenator but changed to a bubble oxygenator. He worked diligently on the project, using all available time while carrying on his clinical responsibilities as a member of the full-time surgical staff.

By the early 1950s, the Professor was aware that the lead in further advancement in the field of cardiovascular surgery was being taken by other institutions and individuals; needless to say, he was not happy about it. Much had been accomplished in the treatment of cardiac diseases by the use of "blind" techniques. So much more could be accomplished, so many life-saving techniques developed, if one could see what he was doing. Many problems simply could not be corrected blindly. This meant the perfection of an artificial circulation, a heart-lung machine that would take over the function of the heart and lungs while the heart was opened for surgery. By the mid-1950s, with no open-heart procedures being performed on his service, Dr. Blalock decided that Hopkins must make progress in cardiovascular surgery. He felt that the man for the job—deeply interested, extremely capable, and well prepared for the task—was on his staff. He assigned the responsibility for the development of a program for open-heart surgery to Dr. Bahnson. He also asked Dr. Frank Spencer, who just completed his residency, to work with him. After years of conscientious effort, in March 1956 they performed their first open-heart procedure with the use of a heart-lung machine that incorporated the DeWall bubble oxygenator. After twenty-seven cases, they changed to a screen oxygenator developed and described as a "Simplified Pump Oxygenator with Flow Equal to Normal Cardiac Output" by Kay and Gaertner.[55] The machine was built in the shop of the department of surgery by Jack Edwards, a machinist.

Dr. Robert A. Gaertner was spending two years during his surgical training at the National Heart Institute, where Dr. Kay had gone on completion of his residency in 1954. Gaertner completed his training as resident in surgery in 1960. He had also worked in the Hunterian Laboratory, where he had performed studies on experimental coarctation of the ascending aorta in collaboration with Dr. Blalock.[56]

During the process of integrating the schedule of open-heart procedures with routine closed procedures, Blue Baby operations, and resections of coarctation of the aorta, Dr. Blalock did not actively participate in the open-heart procedures. A few of the closed procedures were being performed by others; thus he had more time to be in the laboratory, although he never participated in the actual work. Noticing his obvious change of pace, I commented about it to him. His reply was, "Let's face it Vivien, we're getting older. These young fellows can do a much better job than I can. There's no point in my beating myself out with them around. They're good."

Dr. Bahnson left Hopkins in 1962 to become Professor and Chairman of Surgery at the University of Pittsburgh, a post he still holds. Frank Spencer went to the University of Kentucky at Lexington as Professor in the Department of Surgery and is now Professor and Chairman of the Department of Surgery at New York University.

Medical doctors, as well as civilians, were still subject to the military draft in the mid-1950s, even though World War II had been over for some years. Military service credit was given to doctors who spent time in the National Health Institutes. It was not unusual for the young doctors in training to spend two years, during or immediately upon completion of their residency, at the National Institutes of Health (NIH), the National Heart Institute, or Walter Reed Army Medical Center either in research or clinical activity.

David C. Sabiston, Jr., a medical student who had worked with me in the laboratory one summer, received his M.D. degree from Hopkins in 1947. He proceeded with his surgical training, completing his residency in 1953. To fulfill his obligation to the military, Dr. Sabiston spent the two years following completion of his residency with Dr. Donald E. Gregg in his research laboratory at Walter Reed Army Medical Center. His laboratory experience put him in good stead when he returned to Hopkins and the full-time surgical staff in 1955. Dr. Blalock had taken a special liking to Dr. Sabiston and adopted him as "one of his boys," a relationship they both enjoyed.

Because the new, young full-time staff members had few responsibilities during the first several months of their tenure, Dr. Sabiston was able to work in the laboratory. Dr. Jean P. Fauteux, a French-Canadian who had graduated from the University of Montreal, was a Fellow in the laboratory in 1955–56, and the Professor assigned him to work with Dr. Sabiston. Sabiston, the serious, conscientious researcher and teacher, and Fauteux, the student eager to learn, made a good team. Sabiston's mien and demeanor around the laboratory soon earned him the title "Little Professor."

At the time, coronary vascular insufficiency was one of the most difficult problems being investigated. Dr. Blalock and numerous other researchers were addressing the problem of these patients who, with compromised coronary circulation, often suffered angina with the risk of fatal coronary attack. Dr. Arthur Vineberg of Montreal had devised a method of implanting the internal mammary artery in a tunnel in the left ventricular wall to increase the circulation in the myocardium. He was using the procedure clinically, but its effectiveness was controversial. Dr. Blalock had me perform the procedure on a small group of animals that we had studied several months later. Most of the implanted vessels were thrombosed, and in only one of them could we demonstrate any communication between the implanted vessel and the coronary vessels by the use of india ink.

Working with the Professor, Dr. Sabiston undertook an extensive and elaborate study,[57] which included a comparison of similar implants in other organs, the spleen, the liver, and the sterno mastoid muscle. The common carotid artery, being of larger caliber than the internal mammary artery, was chosen for implantation into the myocardium. The vessel was freed, doubly ligated, and divided high in the neck preserving its terminal branches. It was pulled down into the chest through an incision in the left fourth intercostal space. A bulldog clamp was placed on the carotid at its origin and the ligature removed from the terminal branches (see fig. 54). A tunnel was made in the wall of the left ventricle with an Adson hemostat. The myocardium was entered at the apex of the heart with the tip of the hemostat emerging at the atrioventricular groove. The tip of the carotid was grasped in the hemostat and pulled through the tunnel and anchored with a silk suture (see fig. 55). The animals were studied at periods averaging four months. In a series of 32 such implants, 28 (82 percent) were found to be patent. Communication between the implanted vessel and the coronary vascular bed was demonstrated in 21 of 23 (91 percent) by the injection into the implanted vessel of Hill's mass or sodium iodide, both radio-opaque materials (see fig. 56) or bio-plastic. With use of the latter material, the entire mass was subsequently digested with hydrochloric acid, leaving a cast of the implanted vessel and the communication. To demonstrate any protective effect the procedure might have, we ligated the anterior descending coronary artery at its origin at the left main coronary artery in fourteen animals. Nine (64 percent) of the animals survived the ligation; the others died within twenty-four hours. At later autopsy of those that had survived the ligation, the implanted carotid was nevertheless found to be thrombosed in one animal.

During his sojourn at Hopkins, Dr. Sabiston worked consistently in the laboratory, all the while carrying an ever-increasing load of clinical and administrative responsibility. His most outstanding work, usually in collaboration with the Professor, was with coronary circulation, and they co-published many clinical and scientific papers. He organized good teams of students and Fellows for most of his studies. In 1957 he hired James Bradsher as his laboratory assistant. "Brad," as he was called, be-

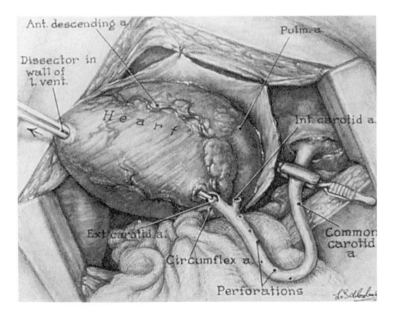

Fig. 54. *Arterial implants into the myocardium—a method used to implant the carotid artery into the left ventricular myocardium. The carotid artery has been ligated and divided high in the neck and pulled down into the chest. The dissector has tunneled the myocardium of the left ventricle and is in place to pull carotid through tunnel. From Sabiston, D. C., Jr.; Fauteux, J. P.; and Blalock, A.: Fate of arterial implants in the left ventricular myocardium, Annals of Surgery 145:927, June 1957, with permission.*

came invaluable in getting various projects set up and in assisting with experiments. Dr. Sabiston always had so many Fellows or students that there was little chance for Brad to become a finished surgical technician.

Among the other Fellows who later worked with Dr. Sabiston was Dr. Lee Riley, Jr., a graduate of the University of Oklahoma who had interned in general surgery at Hopkins. After a year in the laboratory, he concentrated his efforts on orthopedic surgery, completing his residency in that field in 1963. Dr. Riley is currently Professor of Orthopedic Surgery and Director of the Department of Orthopedic Surgery at Hopkins. Dr. James Talbert, a graduate of Vanderbilt University, interned in surgery and spent a year working in the laboratory as a Fellow. He became the first resident in pediatric surgery and is presently Professor of Pediatric Surgery and Chief of the Division of Pediatric Surgery at the University of Florida at Gainesville.

In 1964 Dr. Sabiston was appointed Robert Garrett Profesor of Children's Surgery at Hopkins. He shortly relinquished the appointment to become Professor of Surgery and Chairman of the Department of Surgery at Duke University Medical Center. He was last of the many to be named

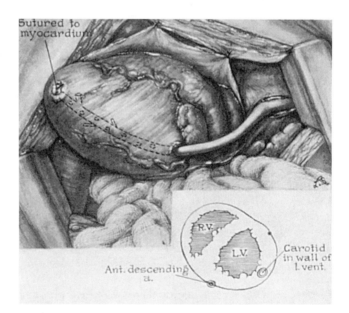

Fig. 55. Completion of procedure illustrating arterial implant in the left ventricular myocardium. Dotted lines indicate the portion of the carotid within the myocardial wall. From Sabiston, D. C., Jr.; Fauteux, J. P.; and Blalock, A.: Fate of arterial implants in the left ventricular myocardium, Annals of Surgery 145:927, June 1957, with permission.

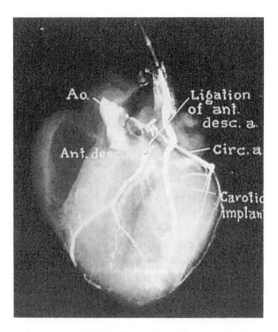

Fig. 56. X-ray of specimen in which the carotid artery has been injected with a concentrated solution of sodium iodide 120 days after implantation. The normal coronary arterial system is well filled and the dye may be seen in the proximal aorta. This animal survived ligation of the anterior descending coronary artery and back-filling can be seen to the point of the ligation. From Sabiston, D. C., Jr.; Fauteux, J. P.; and Blalock, A.: Fate of arterial implants in the left ventricular myocardium, Annals of Surgery 145 : 927, June 1957, with permission.

as head of a department during the Blalock regime. When Dr. Sabiston went to Duke Brad went with him and is now Administrative Coordinator of the Experimental Surgery Laboratories.

In 1962 Dr. William B. Kouwenhoven was awarded the Edison Medal by the American Institute of Electrical Engineers. In his acceptance speech,* after reviewing his earlier studies, he recalled, "In 1951, with the cooperation of the Department of Surgery at the Hopkins School of Medicine and with funds provided by the Edison Electric Institute, I began a further study of the possibility of developing a closed chest defibrillator that would be portable, effective, simple to operate, and the shock of which could be sent safely through the chest of an individual whose heart was beating normally without fear of injury. I believed

*The following words from Dr. Kouwenhoven's speech are quoted from *Electrical Engineering*, p. 5, March 1962, © 1962 AIEE, IEEE.

that such a device might be made a part of the equipment of every line truck. . . . From 1951 on, as our original team had disbanded, I had the cooperation of surgical trainees—a different one each year—and various staff members also collaborated in the work."[58]

Although Dr. Kouwenhoven had the cooperation of the surgical trainees, they did not work with him on a regular continuing basis as had Dr. Kay and I during 1950 and 1951. During that period, a technique for the direct massage of the heart and a defibrillator for resuscitation in the open chest had been developed. Work had also begun on closed-chest defibrillation of the heart. Dr. Kouwenhoven was still active on Homewood campus as Dean of the School of Engineering and Chairman and Professor of Electrical Engineering, posts he held until 1954. While spending part of his time in the laboratory at the Medical School, he was also lecturing at Homewood, a very busy schedule for a man who had celebrated his sixty-fifty birthday in 1951. Among the many individuals who collaborated with him on his continuing studies were Dr. William Milnor of the regular faculty; Mr. Douglas Clark, a Fellow in Surgery from Glasgow, Scotland; Dr. William R. Chestnut, a Fellow in Medicine; and Dr. Frederick Mugler, a Fellow in Cardiology. Dr. Kouwenhoven (see fig. 57) had an undergraduate student, G. Guy Knickerbocker, working with him on various projects at Homewood. Upon graduation in 1954, Knickerbocker continued to work at Homewood but began coming to the laboratory to assist Dr. Kouwenhoven. In the fall he began postgraduate studies while continuing to work in the laboratory.

Dr. Kouwenhoven's interest in all phases of the effects of electric currents, regardless of the origin, led to studies on the dangers of capacitor discharge in television sets. Most of his effort in the laboratory, however, was spent establishing fibrillating parameters of 60-Hz alternating current. By early 1957, after hundreds of experiments, sufficient data had been collected to establish an electric shock time of ¼ second of a 480-volt current to externally defibrillate the heart of an adult and 240 volts for a small child. An external defibrillator unit (see fig. 58) was built for the Johns Hopkins Hospital[59] and was first used on a patient on March 28, 1957. The unit was not portable, and electric current was supplied by standard 120-volt AC electric lines. Instructions with the unit stated that if the defibrillated heart is to resume a normal beat spontaneously, defibrillation must be applied promptly, preferably within two minutes of the onset of fibrillation. This meant that such a unit had to be immediately available. For the patient in bed with the electrocardiogram being monitored, the two-minute time limit might suffice, but for the fully clothed person who collapses in a hospital corridor, this may not allow sufficient time.

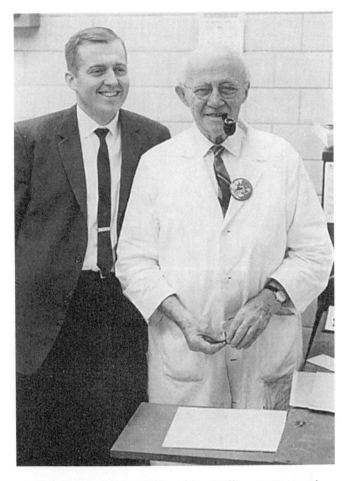

Fig. 57. G. Guy Knickerbocker (left) with Dr. William B. Kouwenhoven (right), c. 1960, whose work on electrical defibrillation of the heart has saved an untold number of lives. Knickerbocker found that the heart could be massaged externally until the defibrillating shock could be administered.

Dr. Kouwenhoven went back to the laboratory, concentrating on the use of capacitors, in which the required electrical charge could be stored and carried into the field where the linemen worked. To save the time required in lowering a victim to the ground, a unit was envisioned that could be strapped to the back of the rescuer and carried up the power pole to defibrillate the victim of electric shock, who is usually held by his safety belt at or near the top of the pole. Numerous experiments on external defibrillation had shown that if sufficient pressure was not applied to

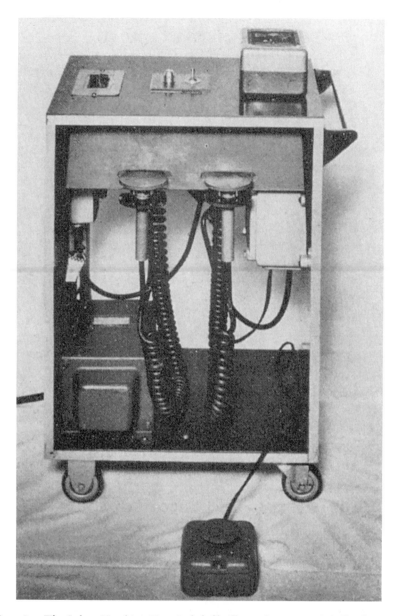

Fig. 58. *The Johns Hopkins Hospital defibrillator for external defibrillation of the heart was developed as the result of hundreds of experiments carried out by Dr. William B. Kouwenhoven and his research team. From Kouwenhoven, W. B.; Milnor, W. R.; Knickerbocker, G. G.; and Chestnut, W. R.: Closed chest defibrillation of the heart,* Surgery *42(3):550, September 1957, with permission.*

the defibrillator electrodes to assure adequate contact when placed on the chest, the effect of the defibrillating shock would be compromised. To enable a single rescuer to apply sufficient pressure on the electrodes and administer the defibrillating shock, switches, with strong springs requiring eight to ten pounds of pressure to trip, would have to be placed within the handles of the two electrodes.

Knickerbocker, by then working full time in the laboratory, was fully aware of the requirement of pressure on the electrodes. He did many of the experiments, even in Dr. Kouwenhoven's absence and sometimes with the assistance of a medical student. He was young, vigorous, conscientious, and observant. To avoid compromising the effect of the defibrillating shock, he applied the electrodes with such force that a pulselike wave appeared on the screen that monitored blood pressure and electrocardiogram. He was impressed by this and wondered if by compressing the chest wall he could sufficiently massage the heart to force circulation of the blood. If this was possible, he wondered if he could extend the two-minute limit on administration of the defibrillating shock after the onset of fibrillation. Having tried it on several occasions and feeling fairly certain that he could, he informed Dr. Kouwenhoven.

In the mid-1950s, James R. Jude, an assistant resident, was performing experiments related to the use of hypothermia in cardiac surgery. Ventricular fibrillation is often encountered in hypothermia, and Kouwenhoven and Knickerbocker had collaborated with Jude in defibrillating the hearts of experimental animals. Jude spent two years with the Glenn Morrow group at the National Institutes of Health in Bethesda but continued some research in the laboratory, commuting on weekends. Knickerbocker kept in fairly close contact with him and discussed the experiment he was performing on the closed-chest massage of the heart.

A research project may become monotonous when the performance of a procedure becomes routine. If this occurs, one tends to lose perspective of the overall problem and little thought is given to alternate approaches to its solution. In this event, it is wise to turn to another project for diversion, which may have been Dr. Blalock's reason for investigating several problems simultaneously. In Dr. Kouwenhoven's laboratory, the same philosophy seemed to prevail. While Dr. Kouwenhoven was on a trip to Europe, Knickerbocker was performing experiments that were indirectly related to the problem of fibrillation. However, one of his experimental animals went into ventricular fibrillation and his immediate reaction was to begin intermittent compressions of the chest. Looking around, he found that there was no defibrillator in the laboratory. He instructed the medical student working with him to continue the intermittent compression of the chest while he went to the EKG laboratory, located several floors below. Returning to his laboratory with an apparatus, he administered the defibrillating shock. The animal recovered completely. Knickerbocker was not working directly on a solution to the problem of external defibrillation of the heart, but he was convinced of the efficacy of external cardiac massage. On Dr. Jude's return from Bethesda, Dr. Blalock assigned him as a physician to work with William B. Kouwenhoven, Dr. Ing, and G. Guy Knickerbocker, B.S., and to clinically evaluate their experiments on external cardiac massage.

Upon moving into the new laboratory facilities on the hospital grounds in 1955, Dr. Blalock had instituted a research conference. These monthly conferences were held in the classroom area of the Surgical Research Laboratory at 1 p.m., after the Professor's Friday noon clinic. Progress reports of the ongoing research projects were presented and discussed. After the work on external cardiac massage was presented, the Professor voiced an opinion he'd expressed many times: The method might work on children, but he doubted that sufficient excursion of the chest wall could be obtained in adults for it to be effective. He turned to Lee Riley, a Fellow working with Sabiston, and said, "I don't think that will work, do you?" Not being prepared to defend a different point of view, even though familiar with the project, Riley sheepishly replied "No Sir." Henry Bahnson first used the method successfully to resuscitate a two-year-old child in February 1958. Later the same year, Jude used it to resuscitate a forty-year-old woman. Although he'd been skeptical, the Professor was proud of Dr. Kouwenhoven and his team, and of the fact that the technique would work in adults as well as children. He was particularly pleased that the work had come from his laboratory.

James O. Elam, M.D., and Peter Safar, M.D., of the faculty in Anesthesiology, had perfected the mouth-to-mouth method for forced ventilation of the lungs. By combining artificial respiration and intermittent pressure to the lower sternum, sufficient pressure is applied to the heart to circulate enough oxygenated blood to maintain life until a defibrillating shock can be administered, possibly an hour or more. The combined procedures produced the currently well-established and widely used method known as cardiopulmonary resuscitation or simply CPR. The method was taught to the Baltimore ambulance crews by Drs. Kouwenhoven, Jude and Knickerbocker beginning in 1959 and has been adopted by ambulance crews in many cities. The Red Cross is also teaching this method of resuscitation to laymen. The defibrillator unit, now standard equipment in all modern hospitals, has saved the lives of an untold number of people. Dr. Jude is presently Professor of Surgery at the University of Miami. Knickerbocker, having received a Ph.D. in bioengineering from

Hopkins in 1970, is Chief Scientist at the Emergency Care Research Institute in Philadelphia.

In view of advanced technology and analytical methods available in 1960, Dr. Blalock had Dr. James Isaacs and me prepare several animals with transplanted adrenals for study. The adrenal gland had first been transplanted to the neck in 1939 at Vanderbilt, and there was no doubt about its viability. The other adrenal had been removed and the animal would have died witnn five days in the absence of some functional adrenal cortical tissue to produce the cortical steroid hormone. In these animals with transplants, the external jugular vein lies just beneath the skin. The vein contains only the blood returning from the transplanted adrenal gland, making it an ideal preparation from which to obtain blood to be analyzed for adrenal function. In bioassay of blood thus obtained, in 1939 we could not clearly demonstrate the presence of epinephrine even though medullary cells appeared on histological sections. Studies of these animals by Dr. Isaacs and Dr. Claude Migeon, the endocrinologist who is now Professor of Pediatrics at Hopkins, confirmed the functioning of the adrenal cortex by its production of corticosteroid hormone. The lack of catecholamines in their assays indicated that the medulla of the adrenal did not survive the transplantation.[60]

Dr. Isaacs, a fully trained surgeon having completed his residency in 1957, was deeply interested in biochemistry. He talked of trace metals and their importance and function in body chemistry, of DNA when it had barely been recognized, and of the many endocrine and biochemical factors in human physiology. On one occasion, he gave Dr. Blalock and me quite a long discourse on the subject. When he left, Dr. Blalock turned to me, smiled, and asked, "Do you have any idea what that fellow is talking about?"

On one occasion, I was demonstrating a procedure that Dr. Blalock knew of but had not seen performed. Until the demonstration I'd had no difficulty, but this time nothing went right. At one point I remarked that Murphy's Law was at work and continued with the procedure. About fifteen minutes later, the Professor was leaving but turned to ask, "Oh! What is Murphy's Law?" It was difficult not to laugh. I replied, "If anything can go wrong, it will." He smiled faintly and walked away. There were numerous versions of Murphy's Law that had been going around the laboratory for several years and I was amused that he obviously had not heard any of them.

During my years of work in the laboratory, I'd made numerous attempts, many of which went unrecorded. How numerous these attempts were became more apparent as time passed. In discussing upcoming projects with the younger Fellows and researchers, I often found that I'd had experience with the ideas they would present. For years I spoke freely of my experiences with the problems they proposed, and the pitfalls and difficulties I'd encountered. It was often discouraging. Then some years ago I heard a story. I can neither recall its origin nor attest to its validity, but I think it demonstrates an important point. Aeronautical engineers have devised a formula establishing a given ratio of wing surface area to fuselage or body surface area for the body to become buoyant and fly. The bumblebee, with his large body and relatively small wings, in no way conforms. According to the formula, it is impossible for him to fly. The engineers, however, haven't gotten the word to the bumblebee so he goes on his merry way, flying. After hearing this story, in order not to discourage anyone, I became very reserved in relating my experiences—others might succeed where I had failed.

18

In 1957 a news item appeared in *The Baltimore News–Post* (December 14) and *Time* (December 23). Both carried a picture of a dog being examined postoperatively. The *Time* article states that Surgeon Blalock repaid part of the debt he owed to dogs for their use in perfecting the Blue Baby operation; the dog, a Rottweiler pup named Squeaky had been suspected of having a heart defect, but examination by Blalock and pediatrician Helen Taussig showed that the trouble was intestinal blockage from an auto accident. Decision: immediate surgery performed by Surgeon Blalock with an operating time of 1½ hours. In the other article the legend identifies the examiner as an operating-room aide and states that Squeaky, owned by Mrs. Geraldine Carter, could some day tell her pups, "Darlings, your mother got operated on by Dr. Alfred Blalock."

The actual story is as follows. The day before the arrival of Mrs. Carter in the laboratory, Dr. Blalock had informed me that she was coming to bring her pup, which she thought surely must have a congenital heart defect because of the episodes of dyspnea and cyanosis. He had told me to see if I could find out what was wrong with her dog. When Mrs. Carter arrived with her pet, I asked several questions about the dog and seated her in my office while I carried the "patient" into the laboratory for some routine physical examinations. There was no doubt about the respiratory distress but on auscultation, the heart sounds did not indicate a cardiac problem. Dr. Gardner Smith, identified in the news articles as "a Blalock aide" and as "a laboratory aide," was a Fellow in surgery in the laboratory. He was quite interested and assisted in the examinations and diagnosis. On X-ray, it was determined that the right chest contained something more than an air-filled lung. There was no air in the right chest, and a diaphragmatic hernia was suspected. On further questioning of Mrs. Carter, it was learned that her pet had been struck by an automobile several weeks earlier. When the Professor arrived, I informed him that we thought the dog had a diaphragmatic hernia. He simply asked, "Are you going to fix it?" With the assistance of Dr. Smith, I proceeded to repair the hernia. Dr. Blalock stood by looking over our shoulders until we were near completion of the operation. Gardner W. Smith, M.D., is Professor of Surgery and Deputy Director, Section of Surgical Sciences at Johns Hopkins.

This was not the first unusual occurrence in the laboratory. Before my arrival, Friday afternoons had been set aside for a veterinary clinic, at which time surgery was performed on animals brought in by veterinarians or the public. The operations were usually performed by the Fellows and the procedures were widely varied, from the removal of a simple skin tumor to the enucleation of an eye, repair of a chronic dislocation of a hip, a caesarean section, a mastectomy, a herniorrhaphy, and other procedures. It was excellent experience for the Fellows. Dr. Cushing had started the clinic in part because of the early interest in veterinary pathology. The fees, usually a nominal $5, were put into a fund that, at Christmas, was distributed among Tom Satterfield, Mrs. Dorman, and the other laboratory personnel. The service was free to many of the elderly in the neighborhood who could not afford the fee. Tom said they kept fairly close tabs on the number of cases handled in order to estimate their Christmas bonus. I continued the practice to a limited degree, scheduling procedures only when I had time.

In 1949 Harold F. Burton, a young veterinarian, took over Towson Veterinary Hospital from Dr. John D. Gadd, who was a friend of the laboratory personnel. At the beginning, Dr. Burton visited the laboratory frequently, observing operative procedures being performed by me and by others. He was interested in learning to perform surgery to a greater extent than had been taught in his veterinary school. He negotiated with us about the possibility of taking our course in operative (dog) surgery and was allowed by Dr. Hanlon to fill fourth place on a team of three medical students. I also began to perform surgery at his hospital on some of his more difficult cases, such as repair of diaphragmatic hernia. One of his canine patients with pyometritis appeared so pregnant that she seemed to be two weeks past term. A successful total hysterectomy was performed. I would take sterile supplies and instruments and, if required, a respirator from the laboratory and perform these procedures at night. I found this type of moonlighting quite profitable, as the fees charged by Burton usually far exceeded a week's pay in the laboratory. Burton proceeded to secure supplies and instruments for his operating room and, of course, become proficient in performing major veterinary surgical procedures.

I was also resident surgeon to the pets of numerous members of the Hopkins faculty and staff. I had established a "private practice" to the extent that my activities came under scrutiny and I was up for discussion in a meeting of the local veterinary association. Fortunately, I had a friend in the organization. Dr. Burton came to my defense, telling them he doubted that any of them could perform the procedures he'd seen me perform and that working full time in the laboratory, I was not likely to damage anyone's practice, whether or not I was a licensed veterinarian. The matter was dropped. For years, Burton and I had an unwritten consultation agreement. If I had a veterinary problem in our kennel, I would consult him. If he had a surgical problem, he would call me.

By fall 1963 we were in a state of winding down and closing out all of Dr. Blalock's research. The process had been going on for at least a year, since no major projects were forthcoming and he would retire in less than a year. About two years earlier, he'd expressed the desire to get some good project under way. I'd told him then that I thought he'd been fortunate to have hit the jackpot twice (the treatment of shock and the Blue Baby operation), something that few people ever accomplish. Dr. Blalock felt he had not received proper credit for his work on shock. In 1964 he wrote that the experimental work of the 1930s was corroborated to a considerable extent in the treatment of the wounded in World War II, that large quantitites of blood, blood substitutes, and plasma expanders were used when indicated.[61]

For the past several years many "feeler experiments," what we hoped would be pilot studies for major projects, had been done but nothing ever came of them. There was seldom a day that research wasn't being done, but nothing that we were very enthusiastic about. Discussions about possible projects were longer, while both of us tended to philosophize and solve or not solve any problem we discussed. This went on to a point that he once remarked, "Damn it, Vivien, we must be getting old. We talk ourselves out of doing anything. Let's do things like we used to and find out what happens."

I hadn't been particularly concerned about the slow-down in our research program. The administrative responsibilities had grown over the years as the amount of research and the number of people involved had increased. I'd become a general consultant to all the investigators and their technicians. Seemingly, there was always some discussion concerning their projects or some specific question to be answered. For some years there had been a minimum of four to six prime investigators with their full-time Fellows and at least an equivalent number of technicians or laboratory assistants. As a result I'd been working under quite a bit of pressure to take care of the administrative responsibilities and consultations and to keep Dr. Blalock's research program going. This slow-down allowed me to work at a more comfortable pace.

On one of his visits during this period I commented that he must be making plans for his retirement the following year. He told me that he'd already received a number of invitations from several departments around the country. When I asked where, he wouldn't specify, but I assumed that with the number of men he'd sent out as chiefs of surgery and chairmen of departments of surgery there'd been many invitations and he'd have difficulty deciding which to accept. He finally said he didn't have any idea as to what he would do. I told him I didn't know what his feelings were in the matter, but I preferred that he not include me in any plans he might consider. I thought he should be in a completely free and independent position in making his plans; I felt just as independent as I had in our earlier years and preferred to be left on my own.

No one had any idea at that time as to who would succeed him. He thanked me and said that the chances were that I would stay on at Hopkins regardless of who was named to fill the position. He added that if I didn't stay, I could probably write my own ticket wherever I wanted to go. I thanked him for the compliment but told him I'd been at Hopkins so long that I didn't know what was going on in the outside world.

The announcement of the appointment of Dr. George D. Zuidema to succeed Dr. Blalock as Chief of Surgery of The Johns Hopkins Hospital and Chairman of the Department of Surgery to Johns Hopkins University was made on February 12, 1964. Dr. Blalock voiced his displeasure about the appointment and I reminded him that his own appointment to the position had not been too well received. Dr. Zuidema had received his surgical training at Massachusetts General Hospital in Boston. He had chosen that institution over Hopkins, to which he'd also applied for a surgical internship upon his graduation from Johns Hopkins School of Medicine in 1953. He had served two years as a research physiologist in aerospace medicine in the air force and returned to Massachusetts General, completing his surgical training as chief resident in 1959. The following year he joined the faculty of the University of Michigan Medical School and at that time held the title of Associate Professor of Surgery. The months rolled by—March, April, and well into May—and I'd heard nothing from Dr. Zuidema.

I began to wonder if Dr. Zuidema might have his own team at Michigan that he would move into Hopkins as Dr. Blalock had done on his move from Vanderbilt. If necessary, I would go to another institution and work for someone other than the Professor. To stay at Hopkins under indirect supervision would put me in an untenable position. I decided to look at other laboratories and find out what my chances of employment would be if things didn't work out to my satisfaction. I could not afford the luxury of several months of unemployment. Claude Brown was quite capable of taking over the laboratory for a few days, so I turned my keys over to him and told him my plans. No one else was told.

I had waited so long that I hadn't had time to make appointments. My first stop was at Indiana University in Indianapolis to see Dr. Harris B. Shumacker, the Professor of Surgery. He had been a Fellow at Hopkins and had briefly been on Dr. Blalock's cardiovascular team. He'd also been on the full-time staff and had done an appreciable amount of work in the laboratory. On my arrival, although unannounced, he was quite cordial. He made changes in his schedule and spent about two hours showing me around his laboratory facilities and other parts of the institution. I related the situation to him and asked about my chances of working in his laboratory. He thought I was unduly concerned and couldn't imagine that I would be allowed to leave Hopkins, but if a problem should develop he would be happy to have me in his laboratory.

My second stop was at Vanderbilt University in Nashville, from where I'd started my career in the laboratory. Dr. H. William Scott was Professor of Surgery and the Chairman of the Department of Surgery. A graduate of Harvard, he'd completed his surgical residency at Hopkins in 1947. Remaining on the full-time surgical staff, he'd done research in the laboratory on cardiovascular diseases. He was called to Vanderbilt in 1952. In March 1954 he performed the first successful open-heart procedure for the removal of an infundibular stenosis and closure of the interventricular defect in a patient with tetralogy of Fallot using hypothermia.

I arrived in Dr. Scott's office shortly after noon, unannounced, and he immediately canceled his appointments for the afternoon. I spent the afternoon talking with him while he showed me around his new laboratory and all the other facilities and buildings that had been added to the institution since my departure twenty-three years earlier. Vanderbilt had grown tremendously, having doubled in size. In midafternoon we drove to his home, where I saw his wife and family. During our conversation, I told him of my concern about the situation at Hopkins. He told me that if any problems arose concerning my position I shouldn't hesitate to come back to Vanderbilt, that he felt confident we could work something out.

Years earlier, when Dr. Scott had received the appointment at Vanderbilt, he had found there was no technician to oversee the Experimental Surgery Laboratory. For some reason unknown to me, Andrew Manlove, whom I had trained, had left the laboratory during Dr. Brooks's tenure as professor. Dr. Scott asked if I would drive his second car from Baltimore to Nashville and try to contact Manlove while there in an effort to get him back in the laboratory. I thought it a good chance for my wife and me to visit our home town, so I agreed. While there, I contacted Manlove and Dr. Scott got him to return to the laboratory. While I was away, Dr. Blalock had learned from Claude that I'd gone to Nashville with Dr. Scott. On seeing me after my return, he whined, "Why did you let Dr. Scott carry you off to Nashville?" I told him of the extra car he wanted driven down and of my good deed in getting Manlove back in the laboratory. His voice calmer, he commented, "Oh, that's all right." Even in 1952 he seemingly hadn't forgotten the trip I'd made to Nashville in 1946 and did not quite trust me to visit there. At this time, with Dr. Blalock only weeks from retirement, I knew he could have no complaints, so the trip had been made a little more leisurely.

On the morning of my return the telephone was ringing when I walked into the office. Miss Cavagnaro called to tell me I had an appointment with Dr. Zuidema (see fig. 59) at 10 a.m. Miss Louise P. Cavagnaro, most often called Miss Cav or simply Cav, had been with the hospital in administration since shortly after World War II and was to be the Administrator for the Department of Surgery under Dr. Zuidema.

On arriving in Dr. Zuidema's office, we exchanged greetings. I congratulated him on his appointment and welcomed him, adding that I'd just made it back in time. He asked where I'd been, and I related briefly

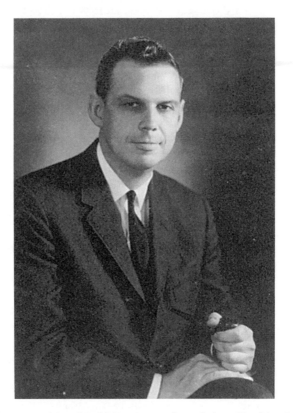

Fig. 59.   Upon receiving his M.D. degree from Johns Hopkins in 1953, Dr. George D. Zuidema turned down a surgical internship at Hopkins. Eleven years later, however, he did accept what he evidently considered a much better offer from his alma mater. He is Warfield M. Firor Professor of Surgery and Director of the Section of Surgical Sciences of Johns Hopkins University and Surgeon-in-Chief of Johns Hopkins Hospital.

where and why I'd gone. He smiled and said that he hoped I enjoyed the trip, but I could just forget it because he'd already included me in his plans and I was to continue running the laboratory. In jest he said that if I had any problems not to hesitate to come to him, that he would be happy to solve them for me. I told him I had only one question and asked where Miss Cav fit into the picture as administrator of the department and what our relationship would be. I was told that she would be in charge of all departmental finances, handling all budgets and grants; she would keep me informed about any funds available for research, but I would be in charge of the laboratory, responsible only to him.

Dr. Blalock had run the department of surgery at Johns Hopkins since his arrival in 1941. In recent years, the major departments had acquired designated administrators. Even though Frances Grebel may have been designated administrator for the department, Dr. Blalock ran the department of surgery. I had not had any direct association with Cav and did not know her except by reputation. The employees and support staff, from whom my information came, considered her demanding, exacting, and a tough task-master. For this reason, I had asked Dr. Zuidema about her position as administrator and my relationship to her. Cav was attractive, with a very pleasant personality. She had been in the U.S. Army Nursing Corps, had seen active duty in Europe during World War II, and had served in Japan after the war. She had retired from the armed services with the rank of major. Her army training and experience had made her officious but at the same time very efficient. I found that no one could hope for a more reasonable, fair, considerate, and pleasant co-worker. Cav knew what needed to be done and how it should be done, and she proceeded to do it without the delays caused by the ever-present administrative red tape. The employees had mistaken her efficiency for toughness. She had more interest in them and their well-being than most of them realized.

The day after the celebration of the seventy-fifth anniversary of the Johns Hopkins Hospital, at which time the clinical science building was named in honor of Dr. Blalock, his portrait had been hung in the lobby. Because the lighting in the new "heart room" (room 12) on the seventh floor of the Alfred Blalock Clinical Science building was inadequate, it had been completely redesigned and installed. In mid-June, about two weeks before his retirement, Dr. Blalock asked me to come to his office on the sixth floor. I was aware that he had recently undergone a laminectomy and had been wearing a brace, but I was somewhat surprised to find him in a wheelchair. We exchanged a few words and he asked that I take him to see the new lighting in the heart room and that on the way out we could stop to see his portrait in the lobby. (I had kept the portrait wrapped and stored behind a large cabinet in the laboratory for about two years.) I took Dr. Blalock both places and then headed for the front entrance of the hospital. Before reaching the exit from the main corridor to enter the rotunda, he had me stop so that he could get out of the wheelchair. Seeing that he was unable to stand erect, I asked if he wanted me to accompany him to the front of the hospital. His reply was "No, don't." I watched as with an almost forty-five-degree stoop and obviously in pain, he slowly disappeared through the exit from the main corridor. When I returned from vacation on September 1, I learned Dr. Blalock was in the hospital. A day or two later I went to see him, but he was asleep. Learning of his general condition from his son William, who was on the hospital administrative staff, I made no further attempt to see him. He died September 15, 1964.

Throughout the Blalock administration, procurement and care of the animals used for research had been the responsibility of the supervisor of the surgical laboratories. During the entire period we had been fortunate in our animal caretakers. On the retirement of Ludwig "Pop" Wolopich in 1956 we had hired Rogers Alston, who was withdrawn, preferred to work alone, and liked animals. There were numerous turnovers in help for him and Pop, but over the twenty-four-year period we had the services of two conscientious, dependable men who assumed primary responsibility for the care of our animals.

The change of administration in 1964 affected the administrative responsibility of the laboratory. A division of animal services had been created within the institution in 1962 and was headed by Edward C. Melby, D.V.M. This group was set up to be responsible for the procurement and care of all research animals within the institution; thus our animal facilities and the responsibility for animal care were transferred to the new division. Being relieved of this responsibility, I anticipated more time for what I liked most—research. I had expressed this in my first conversation with Dr. Zuidema, who had been dubious but left the subject open for further consideration. I felt as if I was being kicked upstairs if I was not to do any research. Dr. Zuidema had a special interest in diseases of the pancreas. He assigned me a problem, but before the pilot studies were completed, I realized I wouldn't have enough time to carry on such a project. It seemed I was stuck with purely supervisory and administrative duties.

In 1965, just before his seventy-sixth birthday, Claude Brown decided to retire after seventeen years of faithful and efficient service in the laboratory. Notice of his retirement was sent to doctors across the country with whom he had worked; as a result, he was presented with a smoking jacket, a box of cigars, and a sizable purse at a retirement party sponsored by the department.

It was not until 1970 that I was able to participate in a major research project. R. Robinson Baker, a Blalock resident in 1961–62, had done a considerable amount of work on the transplantation of organs in dogs and calves. An upcoming project called for the use of baboons in which the entire left lung was to be transplanted. Two baboons were to be done simultaneously, thus each would serve as both donor and recipient. The procedure would require the isolation, occlusion, and division of three structures: the left pulmonary artery and vein and the left main bronchus. These dissections would have to be sufficient in length, after division, to allow for a suture line on both donor and recipient ends of the structures. The lungs were then to be swapped and the ends of the structures matched and sutured together.

This sizable undertaking would require two complete surgical teams. Dr. Baker had a Fellow each year, but Fellows, having had only one year of postdoctoral training, hadn't had time to develop their surgical skills. I felt that now was the chance for me to once again get involved, so I offered to head one of the teams. Without hestitation, Dr. Baker accepted the offer. Working with two separate teams, we performed the procedure on twenty-eight pairs of baboons. The animals in this series of transplants were all treated with immunosuppressives and antibiotics. They represent three sets of studies reported by Baker, Sabanayagam, and others.[62] Dr. Baker is currently Professor of Surgery, Professor of Oncology, and Surgeon in Charge of the General Thoracic Surgical Service at Johns Hopkins.

Part Three

Recognition

19

Shortly after the meeting of the Old Hands Club (former Halsted residents) in February 1969, Dr. George Zuidema informed me that the group had been unanimous in a decision to commission the painting of my portrait. It took a little while to realize the significance of what he had said. My first reaction was that surely I must be dreaming. When my head cleared somewhat, I began asking myself questions. Who is doing this? The Old Hands Club, the doctors with whom I had worked for nearly twenty-eight years. But why did they do it? And what had I done to be ranked with the illustrious whose portraits hung on the walls of Hopkins? Two years later in an interview with Corinne Hammett, who was preparing a feature article for the *Baltimore News-American* covering the presentation of the portrait, she asked the same questions. I gave her the names of some members of the Old Hands Club who may have been instrumental in the commissioning of the portrait so that she could write them for the answers.

George G. Finney, Jr., was in charge of the arrangements for the presentation ceremony. Finney had received his M.D. degree in 1954 and completed his surgical residency in 1959. He and I discussed whether I should make a response. I told him I thought I should, my thinking being that a response would obviate the necessity of writing a note to each contributor, which could be difficult and awkward. My relations with them varied—some were very good friends and others were not. A form letter would not be appropriate, these would have to be individual personal notes. In making a response, I felt that my remarks could be kept general, almost impersonal, and at the same time express my feelings.

The presentation of my portrait was on Februry 27, 1971, as part of the general program of the biennial reunion of former Hopkins medical students, house staff, research fellows, and faculty. I sat with my wife Clara, my family, and a few close friends in the front row of Turner Auditorium, which was filled to capacity. I listened as the presentation and acceptance speeches and remarks were being delivered. I enjoyed all of them, but I particularly appreciated the remarks of Dr. Russel Nelson in his reference to recognition by peers, those who were bestowing this honor upon me. Then came my turn to make whatever remarks I wished. Surely it was my first experience in speaking before such a large and distinguished audience. For almost thirty years I worked behind the scenes. Now I was being brought out front, to center stage with all eyes upon me.

In my remarks, I stated that I had lived with the personal inner satisfaction that I was helping to solve some of the numerous health problems that beset all mankind. I was now being publicly recognized as having played a significant role in research leading to these goals and in the development of the skill of many surgeons. When I'd spoken to Dr. Finney before the ceremony, I'd only had vague ideas of what I would say. In my response I think I covered every facet. Of course, I was elated; it had been the most emotional and gratifying experience of my life (see fig. 60).

Nearing the time for the presentation, I'd begun to wonder where the portrait would be hung. I felt a likely place would be the elevator lobby on the twelfth floor in the laboratory area. Portraits of Dr. Blalock's predecessor Dr. Dean Lewis and of Dr. William F. Rienhoff, Jr., hung there at the time and I concluded mine would join theirs. I had attempted to remain calm throughout the ceremony, but I was astounded when Dr. Nelson stated, "We are going to hang your fine portrait with Professor Blalock. We think you 'hung' together and you had better continue to hang together."

On the following day, Sunday, February 28, I was awakened by the telephone at about 7:30 a.m. The caller was my good friend Leo C. Woods, and our conversation went something like this.

WOODS: "Say, fellow, what's this I see in the newspaper?"

THOMAS: I don't know, I haven't seen the paper, I'm still in bed.

WOODS: Come on, why didn't you tell people what's going on?

THOMAS: I figured you'd know about it soon enough since it would be in the newspapers.

WOODS: Well, if someone was going to put my portrait up somewhere, everybody would have known about it if I had known anything at all about it.

THOMAS: Well, Leo, let's put it this way. This was their show. I didn't have anything to do with it. They handled it, the planning, staging, publicity, everything.

WOODS: How about all these other things you've been doing? Nobody knows anything about it. You haven't told anybody what you do.

THOMAS: If I had been telling you, you would have said I was lying or at least you would have been skeptical. Now you have the chance to read it as they said it so there are no doubts in your mind. You believe it. Now maybe I can talk about it.

Leo, whom I'd met soon after coming to Baltimore, had grown up on the west side of town and as a youngster had delivered newspapers to

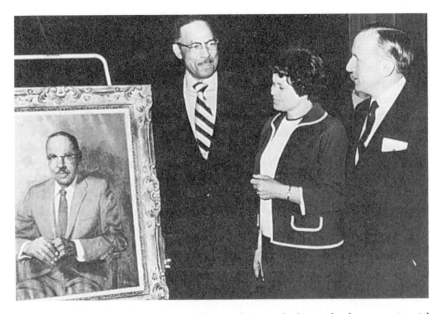

Fig. 60.   After the presentation, Clara and I stand alongside the portrait with Dr. C. Rollins Hanlon, who made the warm and laudatory presentation speech. Courtesy of Afro-American Newspapers.

Dr. Halsted's home on Eutaw Place. He was in the city school system at Dunbar Elementary and had taught both of our children. He received a Master's degree in education from Boston University. He was made a supervisor in the Baltimore school system and retired in 1974, holding the title Specialist in Physical Education.

I received a number of calls that day from friends who were as surprised as I had been when first told about the commissioning of the portrait two years earlier. The presentation was the topic of conversation around the laboratory the following Monday. Dr. Timothy Gardner, a Fellow in the laboratory with the cardiovascular research group under Dr. Vincent Gott, commented and I asked if he'd been there. He replied, "Sure I was there, I wouldn't have missed it for anything. I didn't believe you would be able to talk with all those 'wheels' around." To this I replied, "One thing you have to remember is that I knew all of those wheels when they were small boys like you, many as medical students."

I had worked behind the scenes for nearly thirty years, and after the first year or two no one had given me a second glance. I liked it that way and had been very comfortable in the Hopkins environment. It took quite some time for me to become accustomed to "meeting myself" each morning in the Blalock lobby. Adding to my self-consciousness were the double-takes by visitors and patients. While I waited for an elevator, they would look at me, then at the portrait, and then back at me. I don't think any of the subjects of the numerous portraits that adorn the walls of Hopkins ever regularly stood in such close proximity to their portraits each day. I took it as the penalty one pays for "receiving flowers while one can see them." At first, as a relief, if the Blalock elevator was too long in coming, I would take an elevator in the adjoining Halsted building. I gradually became accustomed to having to live with myself. About a year later, on meeting me in the corridor Dr. Verne Chaney approached with hand extended and a broad smile, saying, "You know, I couldn't believe it when I saw your portrait. I didn't know you were dead, I'm happy to see you back." We both had a big laugh. Dr. Chaney, who was visiting, had occasionally worked with me in the laboratory while a medical student. Upon graduation, he had spent two years on the surgical house staff and three years in anatomy. He is Professor of Surgery and Public Health at the University of Miami and President of INTERMED and the Thomas A. Dooley Foundation.

Late in 1971, a small seven-month-old cat was brought into the office of the Division of Laboratory Animal Medicine, now the Division of Comparative Medicine. The cat had been referred with a suspicion of cardiac abnormality. The owner had noticed that the animal was small, quite inactive, had bluish mucous membranes, and developed seizures after only brief periods of exercise. The seizures had progressed to the extent that the exertion of eating would precipitate an episode.

The cat was seen by Mitchell Bush, D.V.M., then an assistant professor in the division. After extensive diagnostic studies and observations it was concluded that this was a case of tetralogy of Fallot.[63] During the diagnostic process, which extended over a period of several days, I was contacted by Dr. Bush and told of the situation. If their suspected diagnosis was confirmed, he wanted to know if after twenty-five years I was still capable of performing a Blalock-Taussig shunt (Blue Baby operation) and if I would be willing to attempt the procedure on such a small animal. My reply was that even though I might be a little out of practice, I would surely be willing to make the attempt. A few days after the confirmation of their diagnosis, arrangements were made to perform the operation. I asked Louis Jackson, a surgical technician, if he would assist and we prepared sterile instruments and supplies from our laboratory.

On our arrival at Dr. Bush's laboratory, where I saw this patient for the first time, my reaction was much like when I had first seen the patient on whom Dr. Blalock was to perform his first Blue Baby operation. The cat was so small and sick I told Bush that if he could administer anesthesia, I could perform the procedure. I felt it was a toss-up. The cat weighed less than five pounds and was so cyanotic and weak that I doubted it would tolerate anesthesia. Dr. Bush did, however, administer anesthesia and we performed the Blalock-Taussig shunt. The subclavian artery used for the anastomosis was smaller in diameter than that of the comparable vessel in the puppies on which the procedure had been performed. At the completion of the procedure a loud continuous murmur could be heard. Physical activity and appetite increased steadily for seven days and the cat was discharged on the tenth postoperative day.

Dyspnea and seizures began to recur and the cat was readmitted on the thirty-seventh postoperative day. The continuous murmur, indicative of a patent shunt, could not be heard on auscultation. On the forty-fifth day a Pott's procedure,[64] an anastomosis of a small incision in the side of the aorta to a small incision in the side of the left pulmonary artery, was performed. The animal was placed in an oxygen incubator and recovered from anesthesia, but developed marked dyspnea and died eight hours after completion of the operation. Autopsy revealed a quantity of blood in the pericardium and left chest. During the dissection for the Pott's procedure, an inadvertent tear had been made in the pulmonary artery and the resultant bleeding had been controlled by the use of an absorbable hemostatic material (gel foam) and digital pressure. The clot thus formed had evidently been dislodged by the increased pressure in the pulmonary artery. Death was attributed to the hemorrhage. The anastomosis of the subclavian artery to the pulmonary artery was found to be occluded at the suture line.

Many individuals had participated in the diagnosis and treatment of this cat, and many diagnostic methods and types of diagnostic equipment had been used. The studies had included electrocardiography, hematology including bone marrow examination, angiocardiography, and phonocardiography. Those participating in the diagnosis beside Dr. Bush were Daniel Pieroni, M.D., Director of the Pediatric Heart Station; Robert White, M.D., Acting Director of the Cardiovascular Laboratory; Everett James, M.D., Director of the Radiological Research Laboratory; and Dawn Goodman, V.M.D., of the Division of the Laboratory Animal Medicine. Louis Jackson, who assisted in the surgery, had come to the Surgical Research Laboratory in 1965 as laboratory assistant on the cardiovascular research team of Dr. Vincent Gott. Working with Dr. Gott, he had become a full-fledged surgical technician. By this time he was teaching the incoming Fellows many of the techniques of cardiovascular surgery. I could not have had a better assistant.

This era in cardiovascular surgery in the form of the Blue Baby operation had begun as a result of experiments performed on dogs. We had attempted to give the benefits of the new developments to another household pet.

A training program for physicians' assistants, instituted by the School of Health Services at Johns Hopkins in 1973, provided practical training and experience in asepsis, minor surgical techniques, and other procedures that could best be acquired in the laboratory. In the fall of 1974 Elaine Gaze, clinical team coordinator, was referred to me by Dr. Zuidema

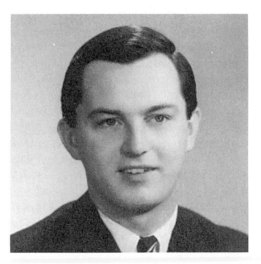

Timothy J. Gardner, M.D.

to organize a schedule and teach what I thought would be most essential and advantageous even though at that time I had no credentials as a faculty member. Students were divided into groups of four, and they were required to attend two sessions. The first session consisted of (1) basic aseptic surgical technique: wearing caps and masks, scrubbing before surgery, and donning sterile gloves; (2) preparing the skin, applying the surgical drape, and performing an intravenous cut-down; (3) controlling bleeding and suturing a full-thickness skin laceration; and (4) performing endotracheal intubations.

At a second session conducted one week later, students would (1) observe wound healing and remove sutures; (2) learn cardiopulmonary resuscitation (CPR) while monitoring blood pressure and EKG, each student participating by performing external cardiac massage; and (3) practice endotracheal intubation.

There were usually four groups; a surgical technician was assigned to work with each of three groups, and I would work with the fourth. The technicians and the prime investigator with whom they worked were Louis Jackson, with Vincent Gott; Jerry Harris, with Alex Haller; and Frederick Gilliam, with John Cameron. James P. Isaacs gave the lecture and conducted the demonstration of cardiopulmonary resuscitation the first year, after which the CPR was done by Robert A. Cordes, Assistant Professor of Anesthesiology. These classes were conducted at Hopkins through 1978, even though the physicians' assistants program had moved to Essex Community College in 1977.

20

In late March 1976, a gentleman came unannounced to my office on the twelfth floor of the Blalock building. When he ascertained that I was Vivien Thomas, he extended his hand and said, "Congratulations." He introduced himself as George H. Callcott of the University of Maryland at College Park. He then went on to inform me that the College Park administration and a faculty-student committee were recommending me to the university's Board of Regents for the awarding of an honorary degree. I told him he must have the wrong person, that it could not possibly be me, to which he replied, "Oh no, we have the right person, we know who you are." He said I would receive a letter in a few days confirming what he was saying. He said that the recommendation to the Board of Regents was a formality and that he wanted to be the first to congratulate me. He gave me the date of the upcoming meeting of the Board of Regents, saying I would be contacted about arrangements for the ceremony. We talked for about fifteen minutes, during which time he asked if I would like to be addressed as Dr. Thomas. I told him I'd have to wait and see. In leaving he said, "I'll be in touch and after our commencement at College Park you will be Dr. Thomas." A day or two later I received a letter confirming what he had said (see fig. 61).

There was no further communication with Callcott until I received a letter dated April 12, 1976 (see fig. 62). In this letter he expressed embarrassment and sadness in having to report to me that the Board of Regents did not approve the recommendation of the College Park campus that I be awarded an honorary Doctor of Science degree. He pointed out that the recommendation had had the unanimous support of the College Park administration and the faculty-student committee.

This news was too much for me to keep to myself, so I decided to show both letters to Dr. Zuidema. When he'd finished reading them he said, "That's too bad, but if it will keep you from feeling too badly about it you had better keep May twenty-first open." He hesitated so long I asked, "For what?" He then told me that Hopkins University was planning to give me an honorary degree. We talked for a few minutes and in the course of the conversation Dr. Zuidema said that there had been "no collusion." Asked if he could be sure of that, he said he could assure me there had been none. Confirmation of this conversation came in a letter

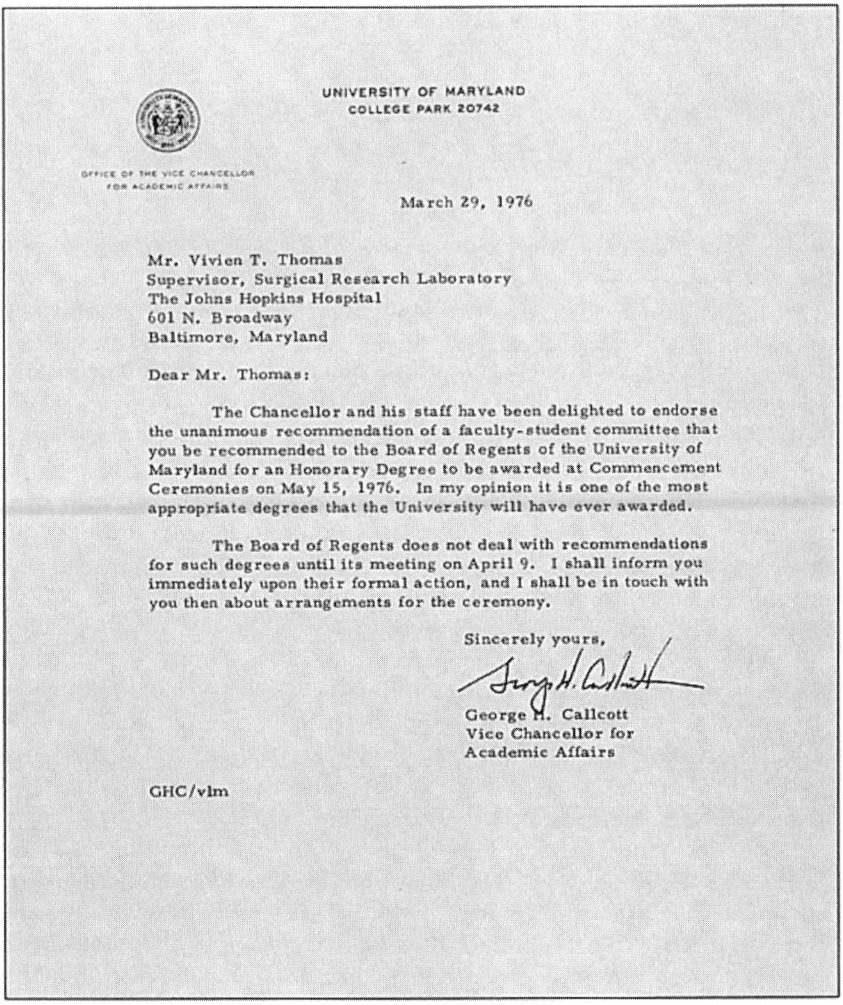

UNIVERSITY OF MARYLAND
COLLEGE PARK 20742

OFFICE OF THE VICE CHANCELLOR
FOR ACADEMIC AFFAIRS

March 29, 1976

Mr. Vivien T. Thomas
Supervisor, Surgical Research Laboratory
The Johns Hopkins Hospital
601 N. Broadway
Baltimore, Maryland

Dear Mr. Thomas:

The Chancellor and his staff have been delighted to endorse the unanimous recommendation of a faculty-student committee that you be recommended to the Board of Regents of the University of Maryland for an Honorary Degree to be awarded at Commencement Ceremonies on May 15, 1976. In my opinion it is one of the most appropriate degrees that the University will have ever awarded.

The Board of Regents does not deal with recommendations for such degrees until its meeting on April 9. I shall inform you immediately upon their formal action, and I shall be in touch with you then about arrangements for the ceremony.

Sincerely yours,

George H. Callcott
Vice Chancellor for
Academic Affairs

GHC/vlm

Fig. 61. Letter from Dr. George H. Callcott, Vice-Chancellor of the University of Maryland at College Park, confirming that I had been recommended by a faculty-student committee to the Board of Regents for an honorary degree.

from President Steven Muller, dated April 16, 1976, in which I was informed that the Board of Trustees of the Johns Hopkins University, upon the recommendation of a special faculty committee, had voted to award an honorary degree at the one-hundredth commencement exercises to be held on the morning of Friday, May 21, 1976 (see fig. 63).

I wrote to Mr. Callcott at the University of Maryland on May 7, 1976, stating in part that "being in the field of research has given me a

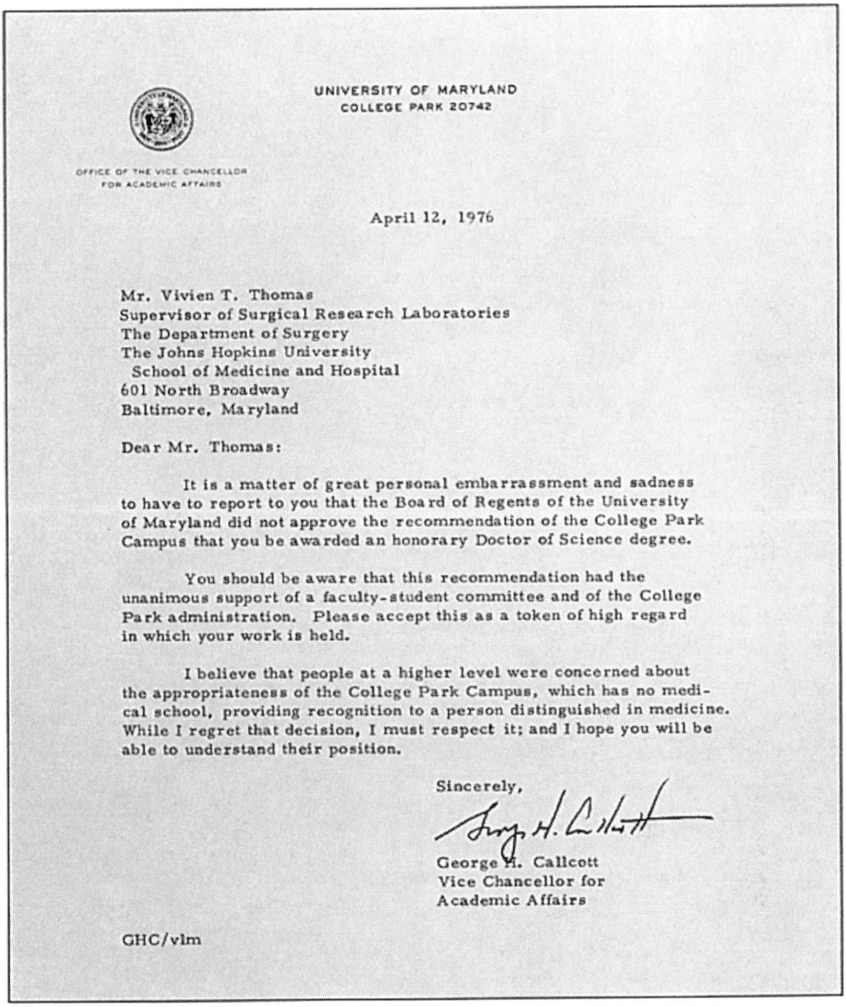

UNIVERSITY OF MARYLAND
COLLEGE PARK 20742

OFFICE OF THE VICE CHANCELLOR
FOR ACADEMIC AFFAIRS

April 12, 1976

Mr. Vivien T. Thomas
Supervisor of Surgical Research Laboratories
The Department of Surgery
The Johns Hopkins University
  School of Medicine and Hospital
601 North Broadway
Baltimore, Maryland

Dear Mr. Thomas:

      It is a matter of great personal embarrassment and sadness
to have to report to you that the Board of Regents of the University
of Maryland did not approve the recommendation of the College Park
Campus that you be awarded an honorary Doctor of Science degree.

      You should be aware that this recommendation had the
unanimous support of a faculty-student committee and of the College
Park administration. Please accept this as a token of high regard
in which your work is held.

      I believe that people at a higher level were concerned about
the appropriateness of the College Park Campus, which has no medical school, providing recognition to a person distinguished in medicine.
While I regret that decision, I must respect it; and I hope you will be
able to understand their position.

Sincerely,

George H. Callcott
Vice Chancellor for
Academic Affairs

GHC/vlm

Fig. 62.   Letter from George H. Callcott, expressing his regret that the Board of Regents of the University of Maryland had not approved the recommendation that I be awarded an honorary Doctor of Science degree.

philosophy about life generally that makes me critical, analytical and somewhat of a skeptic. Conclusions cannot be drawn half way through a research project. If we let our enthusiasm, excitement and expectations rise too high during a project, we may be in for quite a let down when all the results are in and final conclusions are reached. When I received your first letter, I decided 'Let's wait and see.' With this attitude and philosophy my disappointment was not nearly as great as it might have been.

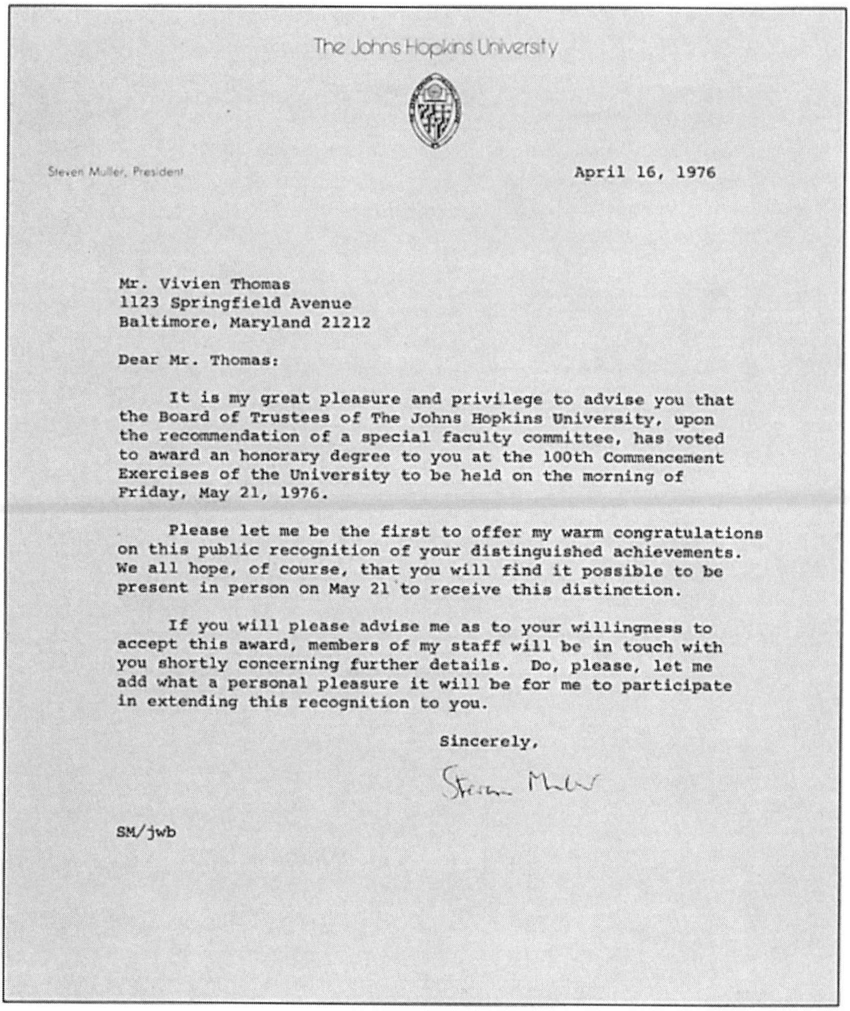

The Johns Hopkins University

Steven Muller, President   April 16, 1976

Mr. Vivien Thomas
1123 Springfield Avenue
Baltimore, Maryland 21212

Dear Mr. Thomas:

It is my great pleasure and privilege to advise you that
the Board of Trustees of The Johns Hopkins University, upon
the recommendation of a special faculty committee, has voted
to award an honorary degree to you at the 100th Commencement
Exercises of the University to be held on the morning of
Friday, May 21, 1976.

Please let me be the first to offer my warm congratulations
on this public recognition of your distinguished achievements.
We all hope, of course, that you will find it possible to be
present in person on May 21 to receive this distinction.

If you will please advise me as to your willingness to
accept this award, members of my staff will be in touch with
you shortly concerning further details. Do, please, let me
add what a personal pleasure it will be for me to participate
in extending this recognition to you.

Sincerely,

Steven Muller

SM/jwb

Fig. 63.   *Letter from Dr. Steven Muller, President of Johns Hopkins University,
confirming that on the recommendation of a special faculty committee to the
Board of Trustees I was to be awarded an honorary degree.*

"My consolation comes in the fact that the Faculty-Student Committee and the College Park Administration of the University of Maryland
did consider and unanimously recommended me for the awarding of an
honorary Doctor of Science degree. To me this consideration and recommendation is in itself an honor."

The news spread around the Hopkins medical institutions, and I was
receiving compliments from strangers as well as friends. Dr. Norman

Anderson, Assistant Professor of Medicine and Assistant Professor of Surgery, had his office and laboratory next to mine. A few days before commencement, I jokingly told him that "Hopkins is really a tough place—it has taken me thirty-five years to get a degree out of them." Dr. Anderson's reply, which I considered among the highest compliments I received, was, "Yes, but look what kind you are getting. That's the deluxe model. That means you have already accomplished something. There are people around here with all kinds of degrees that never have and never will accomplish anything. You've already made a contribution."

I thought that having my portrait presented to the medical institutions five years earlier would have been the full extent of any honor or public recognition ever bestowed upon me. Upon high-school graduation, I had hoped to earn a baccalaureate and a Doctor of Medicine, neither of which materialized. To have an honorary degree conferred upon me was far beyond any hope or expectation I could imagine. Yet, here I was in an academic procession, my first ever, marching with Dr. Milton Eisenhower, a former president of the university, wearing the gold and sable robe of Johns Hopkins University and joining the notables on stage. The ovation on the awarding of the degree was so great that I felt very small (see fig. 64). In returning to my seat on stage, I thought of what Dr. Anderson had said about an honorary degree being the deluxe model and thought that possibly this was the type of ovation that went along with such an honor.

CITATION READ BY HARRY WOOLF IN PRESENTING VIVIEN THOMAS FOR THE
DEGREE OF DOCTOR OF LAWS, MAY 21, 1976

Mr. President, it is with great pride that I present Vivien Thomas, a man who, in the finest tradition of medicine at Johns Hopkins, has richly enhanced the stature of the surgical technician.

Mr. Thomas' ambition when he entered college was to become a physician, but financial difficulties brought on by the crash of 1929 forced him to leave in his freshman year. By a fortunate circumstance, he then answered an advertisement for a laboratory assistant at the Vanderbilt University School of Medicine. He was hired for the job and went to work for a young surgeon named Alfred Blalock.

Dr. Blalock quickly recognized that Mr. Thomas had unusual skills, and taught him to carry out complex vascular and thoracic operations on laboratory animals. Mr. Thomas also learned to perform and to calculate the chemical determinations needed for experiments and to keep clear and precise protocols and records. His extraordinary manual skills became known throughout the school, and in short order, he earned a reputation as an outstanding surgical assistant and research associate, contributing ideas as well as operative and manipulative techniques.

When Dr. Blalock came to Johns Hopkins as chairman of the Department of Surgery in 1941, Mr. Thomas came with him. While the famous

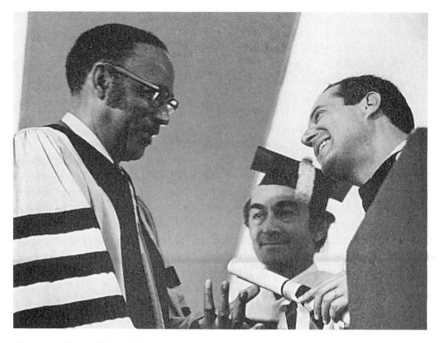

Fig. 64. Harry Woolf, Provost, looks on as the degree of Doctor of Laws is con-ferred on me by Dr. Steven Muller, President of Johns Hopkins University.

Hunterian Laboratory was nominally run by a member of the full-time staff, it was in fact run by Vivien Thomas under Dr. Blalock's direction.

During his years at Johns Hopkins, Mr. Thomas played a vital role in the training of many young surgeons, introducing them to the intricacies of experimental vascular surgery. Virtually every would-be surgeon who passed through Hopkins came under his watchful eye in the laboratory—Denton Cooley, Rollins Hanlon, and among our immediate colleagues, J. Alex Haller, and George Zuidema, to name but a few.

Perhaps the high point of Vivien Thomas' career came in November, 1944, when Dr. Blalock and Dr. Helen Taussig performed the first "blue baby" operation. Mr. Thomas had done much of the experimental work with animals that led to that historic moment, and he stood behind Dr. Blalock as the operation proceeded, offering suggestions and answering questions put to him by Dr. Blalock.

In 1969, a group of the "Old Hands"—former Halsted residents—decided to honor Mr. Thomas by having his portrait painted for presentation to the University and Hospital. At the formal presentation on February 27, 1971, the principal address was given by Dr. Hanlon, then director of the American College of Surgeons. In it, Dr. Hanlon said of Mr. Thomas: "From him I learned the valuable surgical lesson that experimental procedures which seemed nearly impossible to execute when first tried might ultimately be performed with ridiculous ease and economy of time and assistants, after the separate steps had been mastered fully. . . . Vivien Thomas was and is a technician in the finest sense of that term, as all well-rounded surgeons must be technicians." The portrait of Vivien Thomas hangs today in The Johns Hopkins Hospital beside that of Alfred Blalock.

Mr. President, it is a great pleasure to present Vivien Thomas for the degree of Doctor of Laws.

A letter dated January 26, 1977, from Dr. Richard Ross, Dean of the Medical Faculty (see fig. 65), was the result of a conversation with Dr. George Zuidema. The letter informed me of my appointment to the faculty of the Johns Hopkins University as Instructor in Surgery, the appointment being retroactive to July 1, 1976. In my conversation with Dr. Zuidema on June 28, 1976, I had expressed my opinion that, in-

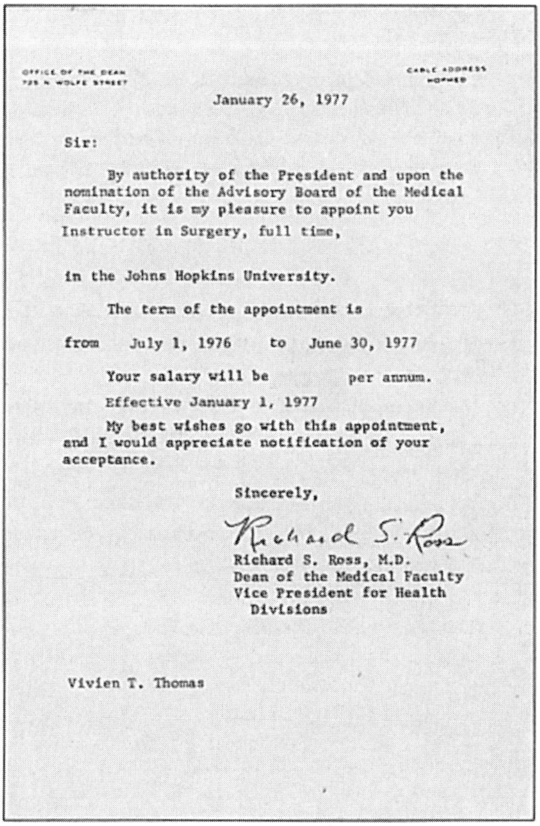

OFFICE OF THE DEAN
725 N. WOLFE STREET

CABLE ADDRESS

January 26, 1977

Sir:

By authority of the President and upon the nomination of the Advisory Board of the Medical Faculty, it is my pleasure to appoint you Instructor in Surgery, full time,

in the Johns Hopkins University.

The term of the appointment is

from July 1, 1976 to June 30, 1977

Your salary will be per annum.

Effective January 1, 1977

My best wishes go with this appointment, and I would appreciate notification of your acceptance.

Sincerely,

Richard S. Ross

Richard S. Ross, M.D.
Dean of the Medical Faculty
Vice President for Health Divisions

Vivien T. Thomas

Fig. 65. Notification of my appointment to the faculty of Johns Hopkins University from Richard S. Ross, Dean of the Medical Faculty.

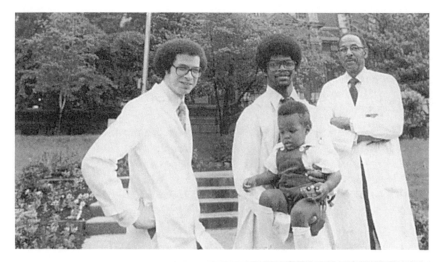

Fig. 66.   Standing outside the Broadway entrance to Johns Hopkins Hospital are Levi Watkins, Jr., who completed his training as resident in surgery in 1978 and is Assistant Professor in the Division of Cardiac Surgery; Reginald Davis, a third-year medical student, with his son; and me, where I had entered 38 years earlier. I retired only weeks after this picture was taken in 1979, taking many memories with me.

asmuch as I had been recognized as a teacher of surgeons, I should be put in that category and serve in that official capacity as a faculty member. I pointed out that I had received the proper credentials from the University for the appointment.

This request for an appointment may have come as somewhat of a surprise, as in two days, on June 30, 1976, I would be eligible for retirement from the support staff. I served in the official capacity as Instructor in Surgery for three years, two of these continuing as supervisor of the Surgical Research Laboratory. I retired and was given emeritus status as of July 1, 1979 (see fig. 66).

References

1. Blalock, A.: Experimental shock: The cause of the low blood pressure produced by muscle injury. *Archives of Surgery* 20:959, June 1930.

2. Daniel, R. A.; Upchurch, S. E.; and Blalock, A.: The absorption from traumatized muscle. *Surgery, Gynecology & Obstetrics* 56:1017, June 1933.

3. Blalock, A.: Acute circulatory failure as exemplified by shock and hemorrhage. *Surgery, Gynecology, & Obstetrics* 58:551, March 1934.

4. Blalock, A., and Beard, J. W.: The effects of adrenalectomy on the cardiac output and blood pressure. *The Journal of Laboratory and Clinical Medicine* 18:941, June 1933.

5. Blalock, A.: The effect of complete occlusion of the thoracic aorta. *The Journal of Thoracic Surgery* 2:69, October 1932.

6. Nystrom, G., and Blalock, A.: Contributions to the technique of pulmonary embolectomy. *The Journal of Thoracic Surgery* 5:169, December 1935.

7. Mason, M. F.; Blalock, A.; and Harrison, T. R.: The direct determination of the renal blood flow and renal oxygen consumption of the unanesthetized dog. *The American Journal of Physiology* 118:667, April 1937.

8. Harrison, T. R., and Blalock, A.: Cardiac output in pneumonia in the dog. *The Journal of Clinical Investigation* 2:435, June 1926.

9. Beard, J. W.; Butler, V.; and Blalock, A.: A study of the effect of division of the cervical oesophagus of the dog. *Surgery, Gynecology & Obstetrics* 53:169, August 1931.

10. Blalock, A.: Experimental studies on the effects of the perforation of peptic ulcers. *Surgery, Gynecology & Obstetrics* 61:20, July 1935.

11. Blalock, A.: Effect of total pneumonectomy on position of esophagus. *Proceedings of the Society for Experimental Biology and Medicine* 32:1552, 1935.

12. Blalock, A.; Cunningham, R. S.; and Robinson, C. S.: Experimental

production of chylothorax by occlusion of the superior vena cava. *Annals of Surgery* 104:359, September 1936.

13. Blalock, A., and Levy, S. E.: Studies on the etiology of renal hypertension. *Annals of Surgery* 106:826, November 1937.

14. Blalock, A.: Successful suture of a wound of the ascending aorta. *JAMA* 103:1617, November 1934.

15. Levy, S. E., and Blalock, A.: Experimental observations on the effects of connecting by suture the left main pulmonary artery to the systemic circulation. *The Journal of Thoracic Surgery* 8:525, June 1939.

16. Levy, S. E., and Blalock, A.: A method for transplanting the adrenal gland of the dog with re-establishment of its blood supply. *Annals of Surgery* 109:84, January 1939.

17. Turner, T. B.: *Heritage of Excellence.* Baltimore: The Johns Hopkins University Press, page 464, 1974.

18. Cressman, R. D., and Blalock, A.: Experimental osteomyelitis. *Surgery* 6:535, October 1939.

19. Cressman, R. D., and Blalock, A.: The effect of pulse upon the flow of lymph. *Proceedings of the Society for Experimental Biology and Medicine* 41:130, 1939.

20. Blalock, A., and Cressman, R. D.: Experimental traumatic shock— role of the nervous system. *Surgery, Gynecology & Obstetrics* 68:278, February 1939.

21. Duncan, G. W., and Blalock, A.: The uniform production of experimental shock by crush injury. *Annals of Surgery* 115:684, April 1942.

22. Blalock, A.: A study of thoracic duct lymph in experimental crush injury and injury produced by gross trauma. *Bulletin of the Johns Hopkins Hospital* 72:54, January 1943.

23. Blalock, A., and Park, E. A.: The surgical treatment of experimental coarctation (atresia) of the aorta. *Annals of Surgery* 119:445, March 1944.

24. Duncan, G. W.; Sarnoff, S. J.; and Rhode, C. M.: Studies on the effect of posture in shock and injury. *Annals of Surgery* 120:24, July 1944.

25. Duncan, G. W.; Irvin, J. L.; and Sarnoff, S. J.: Non-protein nitrogen and protein concentration of serum and cerbro-spinal fluid in shock. *Bulletin of the Johns Hopkins Hospital* 75:135, August 1944.

26. Blalock, A.: Utilization of oxygen by the brain in traumatic shock. *Archives of Surgery* 49:167, September 1944.

27. Hammett, C.: Showcase. *The News-American*, Baltimore, February 28, 1971.

28. Blalock, A., and Taussig, H. B.: The surgical treatment of malformations of the heart in which there is pulmonary stenosis or pulmonary atresia. *JAMA* 128:189, May 1945.

29. Hanlon, C. R.; Johns, T. N. P.; and Thomas, V.: An apparatus for anesthesia in experimental thoracic surgery. *Journal of Thoracic Surgery* 19(6):887, June 1950.

30. Blalock, A.: Effects of an artificial ductus arteriosus on experimental cyanosis and anoxemia. *Archives of Surgery* 52:247, March 1946.

31. Pond, R. B., Sr.: Scientific creativity. *The Johns Hopkins Magazine*, February 1980.

32. Blalock, A.: Stab wound of the heart. *Annals of Surgery* 1931, page 1278.

33. Blalock, A., and Levy, S. E.: Tuberculous pericarditis. *The Journal of Thoracic Surgery* 7:132, December 1937.

34. Ravitch, M. M.: *The Papers of Alfred Blalock*. Baltimore: The Johns Hopkins Press, 1966.

35. Blakemore, A. H.; Lord, J. W.; and Stefko, P. L.: The severed primary artery in war wounded. *Surgery* 12:488, 1942.

36. Johns, T. N. P.: A comparison of suture and non-suture methods for the anastomosis of veins. *Surgery, Gynecology & Obstetrics* 84:939, May 1947.

37. Blalock, A., and Hanlon, C. R.: Interatrial septal defects. *Surgery, Gynecology & Obstetrics* 87:183, August 1948.

38. Schlossberg, L.: *Heart model*. The American Heart Association.

39. Schlossberg, L.: *Mister bones*. The Johns Hopkins Press.

40. Zuidema, G. D., and Schlossberg, L.: *Johns Hopkins Atlas of Human Functional Anatomy*. The Johns Hopkins University Press.

41. Hanlon, C. R., and Blalock, A.: Complete transposition of the aorta and the pulmonary artery: Experimental observations on venous shunts as corrective procedures. *Annals of Surgery* 127:385, March 1948.

42. Michaelian, D. O.; Warfield, D.; and Norris, O.: Genetic progressive hearing loss in the C57/B16 mouse. *Acta Otolaryng* 77:327, 1974.

43. Johns, T. N. P., and Blalock, A.: Mitral insufficiency: Experimental use of a mobile polyvinyl sponge prosthesis. *Annals of Surgery* 140:335, September 1954.

44. Johns, T. N. P.; Sanford, M. C.; and Blalock, A.: An experimental study of the anastomosis of arteries to the coronary sinus of the heart of the dog. *Bulletin of the Johns Hopkins Hospital* 87:1, July 1950.

45. Heimbecker, R.; Thomas, V.; and Blalock, A.: Experimental reversal of the capillary blood flow. *Circulation* 4:116, July 1951.

46. Haller, J. A., et al: *Progress in Pediatric Surgery.* Volume 12. Baltimore: Urban and Schwarzenberg, Inc., 1978.

47. Kay, J.: The treatment of cardiac arrest. *Surgery, Gynecology & Obstetrics* 93:682, December 1951.

48. Kouwenhoven, W. B., and Kay, J. H.: A simple electrical apparatus for the clinical treatment of ventricular fibrillation. *Surgery* 30:781, November 1951.

49. Kay, J. H.; Thomas, V.; and Blalock, A.: The experimental production of high interventricular septal defects. *Surgery, Gynecology & Obstetrics* 96:529, May 1953.

50. Kay, J. H., and Thomas, V.: The experimental production of pulmonary stenosis. *Archives of Surgery* 69:561, November 1954.

51. Kay, J. H., and Thomas, V.: The experimental production of pulmonary insufficiency. *Archives of Surgery* 69:646, November 1954.

52. Kay, J. H.: The influence of cortisone and ACTH on the survival of adrenal homotransplants. *Surgery* 32:686, October 1952.

53. Kay, J. H.; Harrison, T. S.; and Zuidema, G. D.: Effect of sympathectomy on experimental frostbite in the dog. *Surgery* 34:867, November 1953.

54. Pollock, A. V., and Thomas, V.: Replacement of a tricuspid valve cusp by a homologous cusp in dogs. *Surgery, Gynecology & Obstetrics* 103:731, December 1956.

55. Kay, J. H., and Gaertner, R. A.: A simplified pump oxygenator with flow equal to normal cardiac output. *Surgical Forum* 7:267, 1956.

56. Gaertner, R. A., and Blalock, A.: Experimental coarctation of the ascending aorta. *Surgery* 40:712, October 1956.

57. Sabiston, D. C., Jr.; Fauteux, J. P.; and Blalock, A.: The fate of arterial implants in the left ventricular myocardium. *Annals of Surgery* 145:927, June 1957.

58. Kouwenhoven, W. B.: 1961 Edison Medalist. *Electrical Engineering*, March 1962.

59. Kouwenhoven, W. B.; Dr. Ing; Milnor, W. R.; Knickerbocker, G. G.; and Chestnut, W. R.: Closed chest defibrillation of the heart. *Surgery* 42:550, September 1957.

60. Isaacs, J. P.; Blalock, A.; and Migeon, C. J.: Catecholamine and 17-Hydroxycorticosteroid output in dogs with transplanted adrenal glands. *Bulletin of the Johns Hopkins Hospital* 107:105, August 1960.

61. Blalock, A.: Reminiscence: Shock after thirty-four years. *Review of Surgery* 21:229, July–August 1964.

62. Byers, J. M., III; Sabanayagam, P.; Baker, R. R.; and Hutchins, G. M.: Pathologic changes in baboon lung allografts: Comparison of two immunosuppressive regimens. *Annals of Surgery* 178:754, 1973.

63. Bush, M.; Pieroni, D. R.; Goodman, D. G.; White, R. I.; Thomas, V.; and James, A. E., Jr.: Tetralogy of Fallot in a cat. *Journal of the American Veterinary Medical Association* 161(12):1679, 1972.

64. Potts, W. J.; Smith, S.; and Bibson, S.: Anastomosis of the aorta to a pulmonary artery. *JAMA* 132:627, 1946.

Name Index

Subject Index

Detroit, potential move to, 38
Drum, smoked, 20

Embolectomy, pulmonary, 30
Employment, V. Thomas interview for, 10
Esophagus, division of, 33

Fallot, Tetralogy of: development of operation for, ix; early days of operation for, 96–104; experimental studies on, 84–90, 112; genesis of operation for, 36, 39; inception of project, 80–82; role of V. Thomas in early operations for, 91–104
Fellows, in laboratory at Johns Hopkins, 195
Fibrillation, ventricular, 156–60
Fisk University, V. Thomas on maintenance crew at, 7
Frostbite, sympathectomy for, 172

Gloves, preparation and sterilization of, 61

Heart, defibrillation of, 156–58, 199–204
Heart-lung pumps, development of, 194–95
Heart specimens, fixation of, for study, 125
Hopkins. *See* Johns Hopkins
Humane Society, 152
Hunterian Laboratory, 55–56, 190–91
Hypertension: Goldblatt clamps in, 30–31; portal, operation for, 111; pulmonic artery, 36; renal, 38

Implants, arterial, fate of, 196–99
Instrument: for cardiovascular surgery, 74, 96–97, 124; for occlusion of aorta, 74; for occlusion of pulmonary artery, 96; stapler for intestine, 75
Insufficiency, pulmonic, creation of, 165–67
Interatrial septal defects, production of, 118–24
Interventricular septal defects, 161–65; experimental production of, 161–65
Intestine, reversal of circulation in, 149–52

Johns Hopkins: fellows in laboratory, 146–48, 191, 195–96, 198, 200; laboratory, students in, 115, 121, 126; laboratory investigators, 75; move to, 38–40, 49, 53–57; the new laboratory, 184–89; surgical residents, 104, 110,

160; V. Thomas's invitation to, 38
Johns Hopkins Laboratory, student investigators, 74, 110

Kidney: autotransplantation to neck, 34–35; transplantation of, 34–36

Laboratory: cardiac, clinical establishment of, 104–6; catheterization, 104–6; chemical determinations in, 21–22, 32; chemistry, 21–25; equipment, purchase of, 175–76; fellows, 77–79, 148–56; fire in, 189; methods, 23–24, 32; old Hunterian, conditions in, 191
Laboratory, Johns Hopkins: director of, 57–60, 175–76; fellows in, 146, 148, 191, 196; investigators, 75–76, 159; Research Conference, 204; staff and functioning, 55–58; student investigators, 74, 115, 121, 126
Laboratory at Vanderbilt, 10–16, 33–34; expansion of, 21; senior investigators, 16; student investigators, 16, 74
Lung: resection of, experimental, 33; transplantation of, 215
Lymph, collection of, 67

Manometer, mercury, 20
Military draft, 69, 195
Mitral insufficiency, 146–47
Mitral valve, insufficiency, 146–47
Muscle injury, causing shock, 14
Myocardium, arterial implants in, 196–99

Nashville, Negroes in, 4, 43–44
National Institutes of Health, experiments of Blalock trainees for, 194–95
Negro: autobiography of, ix; employability of, at Henry Ford Hospital, 38; housing problems in Baltimore, 57; at Johns Hopkins, 59–65; as laboratory director, 177; in Nashville, 4, 43–47; pay scale of, at Vanderbilt, 44; relations of, to businessmen, 138–39; relations of, to salesmen to, 177; teachers, pay scale of, 43, 45–47
Negro community, reaction to portrait, 220
Nembutal, animal anesthesia with, 27
Newspapers: account of dog operation, 201; interview of V. Thomas, 64